OBSTETRICS AND GYNECOLOGY ADVANCES

IN VITRO FERTILIZATION

OBSTETRICS AND GYNECOLOGY ADVANCES

Additional books in this series can be found on Nova's website under the Series tab.

Additional E-books in this series can be found on Nova's website under the E-books tab.

OBSTETRICS AND GYNECOLOGY ADVANCES

IN VITRO FERTILIZATION

SAMANTHA P. STEIGER
EDITOR

Nova Science Publishers, Inc.
New York

For permission to use material from this book please contact us:
Telephone 631-231-7269; Fax 631-231-8175
Web Site: http://www.novapublishers.com

Library of Congress Cataloging-in-Publication Data

In vitro fertilization / editor, Samantha P. Steiger.
p. ; cm.
Includes bibliographical references and index.
ISBN 978-1-61209-961-3 (hardcover)
1. Fertilization in vitro, Human. I. Steiger, Samantha P.
[DNLM: 1. Fertilization in Vitro. WQ 208]
RG135.I555 2011
618.1'780599--dc22

2011005836

Published by Nova Science Publishers, Inc. †New York

Contents

Preface

IVF is a major treatment in infertility when other methods of assisted reproductive technology have failed. The process involves hormonally controlling the ovulatory process, removing ova (eggs) from the woman's ovaries and letting sperm fertilize them in a fluid medium. This new book presents topical research in the study of in vitro fertilization including management of chronic viral infections in assisted reproduction; posthumous sperm procurement; assisted reproductive technologies for serodiscordant couples with an HIV-1 infection and the impact of laparoscopic ovarian cystectomy for infertile women with endometriomas prior to IVF/ICSI cycles.

Chapter I - Chronic viral diseases impose a special responsibility for healthcare workers devoted to human reproduction to avoid the risk of infection for the partner or the expected child. Attitudes towards carriers of viral infections are rapidly changing as a result of better medication and, consequently, a better long-term prognosis, in which the progress being made in areas of cell biology and biochemistry has contributed. These infections may be transmitted from mother to child at different times not only during pregnancy, but also during intrapartum and postpartum periods.

Gynaecologists should be prepared to counsel affected couples about the risks involved with natural and assisted conception and pregnancy and to recognise available testing and treatment options to optimise outcomes. The authors described the specificities of assisted reproductive techniques for human immunodeficiency virus (HIV)-, hepatitis C virus (HCV) - and hepatitis B virus (VHB) - infected patients.

Chapter II - This chapter deals with intracytoplasmic sperm injection (ICSI) in domestic cattle. Following a brief review on the history of bovine ICSI and the technical aspects of piezo-ICSI, abilities of bovine embryos derived from ICSI and in vitro fertilization (IVF) are comparatively described as recent progress, with special references to active DNA demethylation of pronuclear zygotes, yield and quality of blastocysts, and their cryotolerance. Paternal genome is subjected to replication-independent, genome-wide active demethylation during the early phase after fertilization. Immunofluorescent analysis using anti-5-methylcytosine indicated that paternal genome rapidly demethylated within 10 hours after IVF and 6 hours after ICSI. The demethylation extent in pronuclear zygotes was moderate with $0.4 \leq RM < 0.6$ (RM: relative methylation, paternal methylation level relative to maternal counterpart). Due to the inability of the mechanical stimulation and/or the injected spermatozoon itself to induce proper oocyte activation after ICSI, exogenous activation treatments, such as ionomycin, ethanol, ionomycin + cycloheximide, or ionomycin + 6-dimethylaminopurine, have been applied to ICSI oocytes. Based on a direct comparative study, a new activation regimen composed from two triggers for single calcium increase (5 μM ionomycin for 5 min immediately after ICSI plus 7% ethanol for 5 min 4 hours after ICSI) without using either protein synthesis or protein phosphorylation inhibitors was proposed. While 40% of IVF oocytes reached blastocysts until Day-8, approximately 30% of ICSI oocytes activated with ionomycin + ethanol were able to develop into blastocysts. Such blastocysts were subjected to minimum volume cooling vitrification procedure using Cryotop as cryodevice. Post-warming survival of ICSI-derived fully-expanded blastocysts was similar to that of their IVF-derived counterparts. However, the ability of ICSI-derived expanding blastocysts to survive the vitrification procedures was lower than that of IVF-derived blastocysts, although the ICSI- and IVF-derived fresh blastocysts were of similar quality.

Chapter III- Over 3,500,000 people have been born using Assisted Reproductive Technologies (ART).

This chapter reviews the existing research into the health of this population, highlights uncertainties and attempts to draw lessons for future practice and research.

The introduction of artificial methods to augment an already complex biological phenomenon increases the potential for adverse outcomes.

Much of the adverse outcome relates to morbidity of higher order pregnancies. Early studies were methodologically limited, however as larger, better designed studies and meta-analyses are published it has become clear that ART children have higher rates of preterm birth, low birth weight and slightly higher rates of congenital anomalies.

As existing cohorts get older, evidence regarding longer term biological and sociological outcomes is increasing. Whilst generally reassuring, showing little or no difference in growth, physical health, neurological, neuro-developmental, and psychosocial wellbeing, further research and longer follow up into both adolescent and adult life is required for these and other outcomes.

As newer techniques are developed and become more widespread it will be important to establish prospective surveillance to identify and reduce adverse outcome risk.

Chapter IV – *Posthumous reproduction* is defined as the birth of a child after the death of the father; classically it involves a child being conceived before the father's death and being born afterwards. Posthumous assisted reproduction (PAR) is a form of assisted reproductive technology that involves using the reproductive material of a deceased person for procreative purposes[1]; it consists of obtaining spermatozoa from patients which are either death or in a vegetative state (posthumous sperm procurement - PSP), cryopreservation, and the use of advanced assisted reproductive techniques like intracytoplasmic sperm injection (ISCI) for in vitro fertilization.

Chapter V - The use of assisted reproductive technologies (ART) has been increasing over the past three decades. In developed countries ART account for 1–3% of annual births. The ART developments allow several applications over infertility, for example, serodiscordant human immunodeficiency virus-1 (HIV-1) couples. Many HIV-1 positive people of reproductive age are getting married and wish to have children safely. The use of ART apparently is a viable and safe solution to this problem. This review aims to summarize the current state of the art of assisted reproductive technologies for serodicordant couples with an HIV-1 infection. As fertility care for HIV-1 infected couples is complex it is important to analyze some points. In the 1980s until late 1990s life expectancy after HIV-1 diagnosis was around 20 months, because of such a short life expectancy patients were advised not to get pregnant. Couples with one HIV-1 infected partner had a high risk of horizontal and vertical transmission of the virus, and as consequence they were advised to always use condoms, and if a pregnancy occurs an abortion was indicated. Also it is important to consider the very low sensitivity and a chance of false-negative result of the test available to detect the virus. However, since the application of highly active antiretroviral therapy (HAART), people infected with HIV-1 have been living longer. And in the situation of serodiscordant couples a large body of evidence has demonstrated that the use of assisted reproductive technology, as IUI, IVF and ICSI is effective for active pregnancy, while eliminating the risk of viral transmission. Furthermore, far more sensitive polymerase chain reaction-based methods to detect the presence of HIV-1 not only in blood but also in other fluids including semen had become available. In this review those points will be analyzed with the intent of contributing for a better understanding of this question in order to offer up-to-date assisted reproductive support.

Chapter VI - Knowing what, where and when different proteins are expressed during embryonic development and how functional and structural alterations of proteins control the development programs are fundamental issues in developmental biology. Traditionally, this goal has been achieved by studying one or few proteins at a time, but a research tool that can handle several proteins in parallel would clearly be more valuable. Embryo proteomics is a rapidly emerging research field from the interface of proteomics and embryology that allows simultaneous identification and quantification of multiple proteins in embryonic samples. Besides, embryo proteomic data are essential for the completion of whole proteome catalog of any species because the expression of certain proteins are restricted to early embryonic developmental stages and are not expressed in somatic cells and tissues. Mass spectrometry (MS), applied as key techniques in proteomic research, is providing new insight into mechanism of developmental biology and is expected to improve the efficiency of assisted reproductive technologies (ART). Here, the authors provide some essential information about MS- based proteomics, and their applications to investigate embryo proteome. The authors also discuss the current limitations and measures that can increase our confidence in the accuracy of MS scans used in proteomic experiments.

Chapter VII - Endometriosis is a common, benign, chronic gynecological disorder frequently associated with dysmenorrhea, pelvic pain, and infertility. The prevalence of endometriosis approaches 10–15% of all women of reproductive age while it has been reported that 25–40%of women within fertility have endometriosis. Current guidelines for the treatment of endometriosis include medical or surgical therapies. However, medical treatment has a limited role in the treatment of endometriosis that only offers symptomatic control. Associated with many advantages over traditional abdominal methods, including less hospitalization, smaller incisions, faster recovery time, and faster return to work, the laparoscopic approach for endometriosis has been now widely accepted. Therefore, laparoscopic surgery has traditionally been the standard treatment for patients with endometriosis. Until now, there is no consensus regarding the influence of previous surgery for endometriomas on ovarian function. Some investigators suggested that in vitro fertilization (IVF) outcome is compromised by previous ovarian surgery. Conversely, no adverse impact of prior surgery for endometriosis on ovarian reserve and response to controlled ovarian hyperstimulation (COH) has also been reported. The role of operative laparoscopy before or after IVF in women accompanied with ovarian endometrioma is more complicated. The recent guideline for management of endometriosis in women requiring IVF recommend surgery only carried out in the presence of large ovarian endometrioma. Hence, it needs thorough evaluation in managing ovarian endometriomas for infertile women.

Chapter VIII - Importance of assisted reproductive technology (ART) is being increasingly realized due to progressively escalating cases of male infertility and diseases/treatments affecting spermatogenesis. Currently, sperm is the only choice to restore male fertility through ARTs. However, it may not be possible to retrieve sperm in all male infertility cases such as azoospermia or in prepubertal males who do not produce mature sperm. In such cases, testes-derived male germ-line stem (GS) cells and their in vivo counterpart, spermatogonial stem cells (SSC), have been envisaged as future therapeutic modality for the treatment of male infertility. Indeed, clinical trail of spermatogonial transplantation has already been conducted in both animal and human testes. Here, the authors describe the isolation, characterization and usage of SSC and GS cells in ARTs. The authors also discuss the current limitations in their usage and the possible measures to overcome them. Additionally, alternative methods of deriving sperm from somatic or stem cells have been discussed.

Chapter IX - OMICS technologies (genomic, transcriptomic, proteinomic, metabolomic, and lipidomic) in principle allow visualization of changes that take place when the genetics, nutrition or environment of an organism is altered. Targeted compositional analysis is a valuable tool of assisted reproduction which enables quantitative analysis of biomarkers associated with oocyte and embryo viability. Contemporary embryo assessment strategies are largely based on embryo morphology and cleavage rate. While these systems have been successful in improving pregnancy rates and reducing multiple gestations, their precision is still insufficient. The present chapter describes the current status of embryo assessment techniques for human *in vitro* fertilization and discusses the potential use of OMICS technologies as a predictor of embryo viability.

In: In Vitro Fertilization
Editor: Samantha P. Steiger, pp. 1-33
ISBN 978-1-61209-961-3

Chapter I

Management of Chronic Viral Infections (Human Immunodeficiency Virus, Hepatitis B and Hepatitis C) in Assisted Reproduction

Juan Giles,[1] Carmen Vidal[1] and José Bellver[1,2]
[1]Department of Reproduction, Instituto Valenciano de Infertilidad, Plaza de la Policia Local, 3, Valencia, Spain
[2]Associate Professor. Department of Paediatrics, Obstetrics and Gynaecology, Faculty of Medicine. University of Valencia

Abstract

Chronic viral diseases impose a special responsibility for healthcare workers devoted to human reproduction to avoid the risk of infection for the partner or the expected child. Attitudes towards carriers of viral infections are rapidly changing as a result of better medication and, consequently, a better long-term prognosis, in which the progress being made in areas of cell biology and biochemistry has contributed. These infections may be transmitted from mother to child at different times not only during pregnancy, but also during intrapartum and postpartum periods.

Gynaecologists should be prepared to counsel affected couples about the risks involved with natural and assisted conception and pregnancy and to recognise available testing and treatment options to optimise outcomes. We described the specificities of assisted reproductive techniques for human immunodeficiency virus (HIV)-, hepatitis C virus (HCV) - and hepatitis B virus (VHB) - infected patients.

Keywords: HIV, hepatitis B, hepatitis C, assisted reproduction, pregnancy, infertility

Introduction

Sexually transmitted diseases (SDS), particularly chronic viral infections (human immunodeficiency virus, hepatitis B and hepatitis C), are a special responsibility for gynaecologists given the risk of transmission to offspring [1] or to an uninfected partner [2], and even to other patients [3]. This is why the screening, of these infections before pregnancy is essential for all couples who wish to have children [4], regardless of the way of conception [5]. Clinicians are responsible for explaining to patients the possible means by which infections can be acquired and the advantages of knowing the test result before pregnancy.

Nowadays, specific therapies have significantly improved, which not only allow longer life expectancy and increase the number of couples at childbearing age [6-10], but also permit a lower risk of transmission [11]. In parallel, we have witnessed an evolution of laboratory techniques that have brought about a change in attitudes towards the employment of Assisted Reproduction Technologies (ART) [12-14]. Their use will enable to treat the infertility problems in this group of patients and will help to minimise the risk of transmission.

Nevertheless, ethical conflicts persist [2, 9, 15-17], and very few centres treat this group of patients [18]. Those centres that do not have the resources to offer adequate therapeutic options should refer patients to a centre that follows protocols to manage these patients. Thus it is increasingly accepted that it would be unethical to deny such treatment [12-14, 19].

The current trend is to avoid discrimination and to provide medical care within a multidisciplinary team [20] for achieving a save pregnancy. However, not all Human Immunodeficiency Virus (HIV)-affected couples are good candidates for assisted reproduction. There are cases in which assistance may be withheld, being ethically and legally justifiable to avoid couples in which the procedure is medically inappropriate or involves an excessive attributable risk (e.g., poor health status of the couple or non-compliance) [2, 21, 22].

If one or both members of the couple present an infection which is the object of this review, it is essential to provide accurate information on the potential risks that pregnancy may involve and the available therapeutic options, as well as their limits in each situation. An informed consent must be signed and obtained prior to take any action.

This review aims to cover all the different aspects of conception including sexual transmission, implications for fertility, vertical transmission, current assisted reproduction options, ovarian response in affected women, management of samples in andrology and IVF labs, or techniques to detect viral particles in sperm samples.

Human Immunodeficiency Virus (HIV-1)

For almost 30 years and after 20 million deaths since the first Acquire Immunodeficiency Syndrome (AIDS) diagnosis in 1981, the current number of infected people is 33.4 million *according* to the last Joint United Nations Programme on HIV/AIDS (UNAIDS) [23]. The continuing rise in the population of people living with HIV reflects the combined effects of continued high rates of new HIV infections and the beneficial impact of antiretroviral therapy (ARV) (the total number of people living with the virus was more than 20% higher in 2008 than the figure in 2000).

The percentage of infected females has remained stable for several years at 50%, of whom 85% are of the reproductive age. The number of children living with HIV continues to steadily increase worldwide, although new HIV infections in children appear to have peaked in 2000-2002. This is thought to be chiefly due to HIV prevalence have stabilised among females in general, and to an increasing coverage of programmes broadcast to prevent mother-to-child HIV transmission.

A change in the pattern of infection has been described since heterosexual transmission has sharply increased, and this is the main cause of infection in women in developed countries [23, 24]. Other prevalent groups include users of unscreened blood products, intravenous drug users, sex workers and homosexual men.

The epidemic appears to have stabilised in most regions, although prevalence continues to increase in Eastern Europe and Central Asia and in other parts of Asia given a high rate of new HIV infections. Sub-Saharan Africa remains the most heavily affected region [23, 25].

HIV-2 is less virulent and presents a lower risk of transmission in subjects exposed than HIV-1, and is mainly confined to West Africa. So, we will refer to HIV-1 throughout this chapter as it is responsible for the majority of the cases of infection worldwide.

HIV-1 in Females

The risk of perinatal or female-to-male sexual transmission of HIV-1 is probably associated with viral presence in the cervical and vaginal secretions of HIV1-infected woman and its exact concentration. HIV can be detected in both vaginal and cervical secretions as a cell-free virus or as a cell-associated virus [26, 27].

The most important factor for predicting genital HIV-1 shedding is plasma HIV-1 RNA [28], although it is still detected in the genital secretions of 33% of patients with plasma levels of < 500 copies/ml after receiving HAART (Highly Active Antiretroviral Treatment), and in 25% of women with < 50 copies/ml [29].

Variation of the genital-tract virus level is greater than that for blood [30]. Throughout the menstrual cycle, no statistically significant difference has been observed in the plasma viral load, and no significant association with serum estradiol or progesterone levels has been noted [31, 32]. Other study showed a significant decrease in the genital tract viral load in the periovulatory phase while the plasma viral load remained constant throughout the menstrual cycle [28]. These results suggest that local factors may affect the genital viral load compartment independent of plasma viral load

The presence of higher levels of HIV-1 DNA in cervical secretions has been significantly associated with oral contraceptive pill use, cervical ectopy, and pregnancy [27]. Vitamin A deficiency, gonococcal cervicitis and vaginal candidiasis have also been correlated with significant increases in HIV-1 DNA detection [33]. These risk factors, easily modifiable by simple interventions, may be important determinants of sexual or vertical HIV transmission.

HIV-1 and Female Reproductive Function

HIV-1-infected females are significantly more likely to present gynaecologic disorders. Menstrual alterations have been described in females who present advanced stages of AIDS or lower CD4 T cell counts [34]. Amenorrhoea is associated with both antecedents of drug abuse parenterally and VHC co-infection, irrespectively of the AIDS stage or CD4 T cell counts [35].

A higher incidence of premature ovarian failure has also been reported [36, 37]. Negative factors could be the appearance of opportunist illnesses associated with HIV, a recount of CD4 < 200 cel/microl [38] or drug use [39]. We ought not to forget the endocrine dysfunctions associated with HIV (abnormalities of the pituitary-adrenal, pituitary-thyroid and pituitary-ovarian axes) [40], and the possible effects that antiretroviral drugs (ARV) may have on folliculogenesis, especially protease inhibitors given their influence on the lipid mechanism and insulin resistance [41]. HAART has been significantly related to higher LH, FSH, and estradiol (E2) concentrations [39, 42].

Some studies also reveal a higher incidence of sexually transmitted diseases, with a greater risk of tubal infertility [43] appearing mainly as distal tubal occlusion with hydrosalpinx [44]. The ovarian reserve seems to be affected as evidenced by the aforementioned studies and other recent ones [42, 45, 46], although there are any discrepancies [47].

The results of studies performed in Africa, and also in developed countries, suggest that HIV-1 may have an adverse effect on fecundation and fertility, particularly in cases of advanced disease [38, 48] regardless of the association with STDs [49]. This observation is in line with a recent report of a drop in fertility rates in Europe [50], which suggests subclinical hypogonadism mediated by immunosupression.

Effect of Antiretroviral Therapy in Female Fertility

Access to antiretroviral therapy (ARV) was another key factor guiding the final decision on child bearing [51]. Women are more likely to have antiretroviral treatment side effects, and certain antiretroviral regimens may impair contraceptive efficacy [52]. ARV use is associated with significantly higher pregnancy rates among HIV-infected women in the sub-Saharan Africa, and the possible behavioural or biomedical mechanism that may underlie this association require further investigation [53]. However, data on HAART and fertility in women are limited, so no conclusions can be currently drawn.

In ARV-eligible pregnant women with HIV infection, ARV is a safe and effective means of providing maternal virologic suppression, decreasing infant mortality, and reducing mother-to-child transmission (MTCT) [54].

Lipodystrophy and insulin resistance are well-recognised side effects of HAART. Polycystic ovary syndrome may be an additional side effect secondary to insulin resistance and lipodystrophy [55]. New data, however, demonstrate that common features of polycystic ovary syndrome are not detected among HIV-infected subjects with severe abdominal fat accumulation and hyperinsulinemia [56].

Vertical Transmission

The number of children newly infected with HIV in 2008 was roughly 18% lower than in 2001. (23). Most new infections in children are believed to stem from transmission in the uterus, during delivery or post-partum as a result of breastfeeding; nonetheless in the absence of breastfeeding, it occurs in 35% of cases in the last weeks of pregnancy, and in 65% of cases at birth [57]. Along these lines, a recent study has considered that 50% of HIV infections for non-breastfeeding populations are transmitted to infants at the very end of pregnancy, near the time of labour [58].

Table 1. Risk of Vertical Transmission

Infection	Scenario
HIV-1	- No intervention 15-20% and 35-40% when associated with prolonged breastfeeding - ARV drugs, caesarean delivery and artificial lactation have helped reduce the risk to 1-2%
Hepatitis B	- Acute: 10% when infection occurs in the first trimester and 90% when it occurs in the third trimester. Combining active (vaccination) and passive immunisation (HBIgG) effectiveness in prevention is about 85-95%. - Chronic: 20-30% only HbsAg is positive, reaching 80-90% when HBsAg and HBeAg or the DNA of HBV are positive.
Hepatitis C	- Unknown viral titers: the overall risk of transmission is approximately 5-10% - Females with antibodies against HCV and negative HCV RNA: less than 1-3%, over 4-10% if positive HCV ARN, reaching up to 36% when there are titers > 106 copies/mL. - In cases of co-infection by HIV-1, this risk becomes 10-15%

HBV: hepatitis B virus. HBsAg: hepatitis B surface antigen. HBeAg: hepatitis B e antigen. HBIG Immunoglobulin against hepatitis B. HCV: hepatitis C virus..ARV antiretroviral drugs.

Under ideal conditions, the provision of antiretroviral prophylaxis, caesarean delivery and replacement feeding can reduce transmission from an estimated 30% to 35% with no intervention [59] to around 1% to 2%. [60] (Table 1).

Transmission is greater with high levels of HIV-1 RNA, and is very unlikely in women with a non-detectable viral load or when it is lower than 1000 copies /ml. Nevertheless, the risk of perinatal transmission in women with undetectable HIV RNA levels is possible, and MTCT has been reported among women with all levels of maternal HIV RNA [61]. Additionally, although HIV RNA may be an important risk factor for transmission, other factors also appear to play a role. Therefore, antiretroviral prophylaxis for the prevention of perinatal transmission should be given even to women who have a very low or undetectable viral load on no therapy [61].

Neither pregnancy implies a negative effect on disease progression and survival in well monitored asymptomatic women, nor HIV-1 itself increases the risk of obstetric problems or foetal malformations [62, 63]. The information available suggests that there was less progression of HIV disease, but it was not statistically significant [64]. More recently, data in women who received HAART have also shown that pregnancy is associated with a lower risk of HIV disease progression [65].

However, the newborn of HIV-1-positive mothers present a higher co-morbidity, mainly due to maternal factors such as malnutrition, drug addiction, etc.

HIV-1 in Males

HIV-1 has been detected in the seminal plasma as cell-associated virions (RNA), [66] as well as in the non-spermatic cell fraction of ejaculation as a provirus, mainly in the lymphocitary population [67]. Despite the controversy about its presence in sperm [67-69], other authors have ruled it out [70, 71]. More recently, HIV-1 DNA has been detected in situ in a small percentage of abnormal spermatozoa with a wide range of structural alterations [72]. Their possible role in HIV-1 sexual transmission remains unclear. The latest results indicate that viral DNA is present in purified sperm from HIV-positive men, and that HIV infection of spermatozoa may be associated with lower seminal parameters, as demonstrated by the PCA method (Principal Component Analysis) [73].

Although semen is the main vector of human immunodeficiency virus (HIV) dissemination worldwide, the origin of the virus in this bodily fluid remains unknown. Testis are infected early during the course of infection without association with either any apparent change in testicular morphology or inflammation of the organ. Most HIV-1 RNA apparently originates from the seminal vesicles and prostate because vasectomies did not influence concentrations in semen [74]. The detection of different HIV-1 genotypes in the epididymis and prostate probably confirm local production [75].

Lowered androgen levels have been demonstrated usually, but not systematically, in association with progressive immunosuppression in HIV-affected males [76].

Antiretroviral therapy has also been reported to influence sexual hormones in males [77], and seems to be directly or indirectly related to sexual dysfunction (particularly protease inhibitors) through different mechanisms to some extent, despite the inconsistent results reported among studies [78].

Impact of HIV-1 on Semen Parameters

Although seminal parameters use to remain normal [79], more frequent alterations in terms of number, mobility and leucospermia have been observed in most advanced cases (mainly CD4 < 200 cells/mm3) [80]. Prolonged exposure to asymptomatic, untreated HIV-1 infection does not affect semen quality [81].

An elevated rate of spontaneous abortions has been reported in serodiscordant couples in whom the man is HIV seropositive [82]. It is noteworthy that the majority of these men take antiretroviral (ARV) drugs which may affect semen quality either independently of or in addition to infection.

Genital Tract: A Viral Reservoir

When treatment is absent, the HIV-1 RNA concentration in semen is 10-fold lower than in plasma, although this concentration is higher in semen in some individuals [80, 83]. In general terms, there seem to be no relationship between the male genital tract and the blood reservoir given the different concentrations of virus detected [84], the different genotypes [85], or the variability in response to treatment between both locations. The persistence of the viral release in the semen of HIV1-infected males undergoing ARV is especially significant as they would otherwise show an undetectable blood viral load [86- 88]. Thus when HAART is discontinued, the blood plasma viral load that was undetectable under the presence of the antiretroviral drugs systematically rises again from these reservoirs [89].

The importance of determining the nature of the reservoirs responsible for HIV shedding in semen should be stressed to design more effective therapeutic strategies that can eradicate the virus from semen.

Antiretrovirals for Reducing HIV-1 in Semen

Antiretroviral drugs penetrate adequately into the male genital tract, except for some protease inhibitors [83, 90].Although a parallel drop in the viral load in blood and semen has been reported [20, 24, 25, 86, 91, 92], there may not be a correspondence between them, as previously mentioned, and it appears to be extremely variable among individuals.

The knowledge available about the effect of ARV drugs on seminal parameters is limited; no changes occur after taking zidovudine (AZT), but improvement is noted after HAART [93]. However in HIV-1 patients, further longitudinal studies are required to analyse the impact of the treatment regimen on sperm parameter alterations.

Since concerns about long-term side effects of the antiretroviral therapy have led to postpone its initiation until CD4 counts drop to 200-350 cells/mm3; this scenario does not appear to negatively affect semen parameters [94].

Finally, the theoretical penetration of nucleoside reverse transcriptase inhibitors into spermatozoa or their precursors could result in mitochondrial toxicity and may, therefore, lead to impaired progressive motility. However, this hypothesis remains to be proved [95].

Risk of Sexual Transmission

Worldwide, the predominant mode of HIV-1 transmission is sexual for more than 80%, mainly heterosexual intercourse. Transmission during sexual intercourse through vaginal penetration is extremely variable [96, 97]. The risk of contamination by sexual contact in a stable couple is between 0.1 and 0.5% [98, 99], and is lower than in occasional intercourse [100, 101]. The rate of heterosexual HIV-1 transmission in a population of intravenous drug users (IVDU) is 16% [102].

A recent meta-analysis has suggested that the transmission rate in heterosexual discordant couples from a person on antiretroviral therapy is approximately 0.5 per 100 person-years, while it is 5.6 per 100 person-years for individuals not on antiretroviral therapy [103].

The risk of transmission increases with advanced stages of HIV-1 infection, the level of infection of the viral strain, the viral load, associated genital infections in the HIV1- negative partners, and with the nature of sexual practices [104]. Withdrawal to avoid ejaculation in the vagina had a protective effect on uninfected women, as did the avoidance of anal sex.

Assisted Procreation

Many years ago, HIV-1 infection was considered a serious contraindication to establish a healthy pregnancy. Recent mathematical modelling exercises have suggested that improved access to HIV testing and counselling and to antiretroviral therapy could significantly reduce MTCT [105]. This situation allowed HIV-infected patients to be included in ART (Assisted Reproduction Techniques) programmes to treat their infertility pathologies, to reduce the risk of transmission, or to combine both [106]. No reproductive attempt should ever be made before having done a standardised evaluation of the HIV-1 couple.

Serodiscordant Couples: HIV-1 Positive Females

Recommendations before Pregnancy

In addition to the general components of preconception counselling and care that are appropriate for all women of a reproductive age, HIV-infected women have specific needs that should be addressed [61]. In this group of patients, it is advisable to provide detailed information about the risk of transmission, beginning or modification of ARV therapy, evaluation and prophylaxis of opportunist infections (influenza, Streptococcus pneumoniae, hepatitis B), nutritional state optimisation, and infectious diseases sieving [107, 108]. It is also advisable to perform smear test, cervical culturing, sexually transmitted diseases (STDs) sieving-syphilis, gonorrhoea, Chlamydia and trichomonas-, hepatic function tests, tuberculin and a chest X-ray (if previous ones are lacking) [11, 109].

Assisted Reproduction Techniques (ART)

Despite the low number of available works on the use of ART in HIV-1-infected females, we believe that the risk of vertical transmission is similar to that of natural conception since it happens at the end of the pregnancy and during birth [57, 58,110] in developed countries in which lactation is abolished.

Although several policies have been described, our group believes that only those women whose disease is not advanced with good immune status, such as lymphocytes CD4 ≥ $500/mm^3$ and viral load ≤ $5\text{-}10x10^3$copies/ml, should receive treatment within a multidiscipline frame. If this situation prolongs for more than 6 months and immunological status is excellent, despite the presence of virus in blood, it is advisable to do a resistance test if the patient has previously taken HAART to determine which drugs may be used during pregnancy with a view to reducing the presence of the virus in blood and vertical transmission. After the test, the ART procedure can commence. If the patient has never taken HAART and the viral load is $< 1 \times 10^3$ copies/ml, ART may begin without having to do resistance tests beforehand as it is quite likely that the patient's response to antiretroviral treatment during pregnancy is good [111].

A patient presenting lymphocytes CD4 $< 500/mm^3$ or a viral load of $> 10x10^3$ copies/ml should be sent to an infectologist to start HAART therapy to obtain a non-detectable viral load before starting ART. These inclusion criteria are similar to those that other groups have employed [112, 113].

As regards of the use of ARV drugs before starting ART, different opinions have also been voiced about the viral load cut-off from which ARV should be started, or if this therapy should no longer be administered once pregnancy has been achieved or not [114, 115]. Cochrane's review concludes that ART is a safe, effective means of providing maternal virologic suppression, decreasing infant mortality and reducing MTCT [116]. Specifically the following ARV regimens, Zidovudine (AZT)/Lamividine (3TC)/Nevirapine (NVP), AZT/3TC/Lopinavir + Ritonavir (LPV-r), and AZT/3TC/Abacavir (ABC) have been shown to lower MTCT [116].

Evidently, the indicated guideline will depend on each centre's experience, its follow-up capacity, control of patients once they are pregnant, and the couple's degree of responsibility and commitment under treatment. Moreover, the whole procedure must include an infectologist's advice.

In cases of co-infection by HCV, the viral load to be included in a reproduction protocol should be $< 10^6$ copies /ml since the risk of transmission of HCV below this value drops significantly [117].

According to our experience, it is advisable to perform self-inseminations when no obvious infertility factor can be found. van Leeuwen et al consider that ART should be advised in the case of unsuccessful pregnancy achievement after 1 year in women with regular menstruation cycles [112]. Yet other authors recommend initiating fertility investigation if conception has not occurred within six cycles of self-insemination [118] given the increased risk of infertility (frequency of upper genital tract infections and cervical lesions), particularly in women over the age of 35 [21].

Like other groups, we discourage planned intercourse regardless of the technique used to determine ovulation for the reasons already mentioned [29, 61]. The rate of female-to-male transmission does not appear to significantly differ from that of male-to-female transmission (0.5-1%) [119].

We advise artificial insemination (AI) for self-insemination failure when it is not well tolerated by the couple (they may think it interferes with their sex life), or if a sterility factor has been determined. We used low doses of gonadotropins to avoid multiple pregnancies because premature deliveries could increase the risk of vertical transmission [120]. Another factor that makes the use of low doses of gonadotropins advisable is increased viral load which can be induced in comparison with natural cycles [21].

Some authors do not find the artificial insemination results encouraging [121], while others see no differences with other couples [115]. *In vitro* fertilization (IVF) offers a better pregnancy rate and sometimes allows the transfer of only 1 embryo when prognosis is good. Many groups transfer a maximum of 2 embryos (whatever the patient's age, even with frozen-thawed embryos) [113] because of the increased risk of maternal-foetal transmission with a selective embryo reduction [122], and the prematurity and obstetric complications due to multiple pregnancy [120, 123]. Other authors consider transferring 3 or more embryos under certain circumstances [115].

These advantages of IVF are not associated with a significant increase in risk, although the presence of HIV-1 in follicle fluid has been detected (even in women with a negative viral load) [21]. However, receptors for HIV on the surface of the oocyte itself have not been demonstrated. Theoretically, a viral particle could be injected into a human oocyte during ICSI, analogously to the situation in an HIV-1 infected male [112].

As with all our patients, we use IVF/ICSI or spermatic microinjection (ICSI) in the first cycle to avoid IVF failure since the delay it could cause is more significant in females under ARV who have interrupted it in order to conceive. This attitude is similar to that recorded by other groups [113].

The results available for IVF differ; some authors have found no difference with the general population [115, 124], while others have detected a lower pregnancy rate with own oocytes that disappears with donated oocytes [125] (Table 2).

Ovarian response to stimulation is similar to uninfected HIV-1 women [126]. Other authors found that satisfactory ovarian stimulation was more difficult to achieve (needing higher total doses of recFSH, with longer duration of stimulation and higher percentage of cancelled cycles) when comparing with a non-matched general ART group [113] or with an age-matched group [124]. Because the number of reported IVF and ICSI cycles in HIV-1 infected women is very small, no ultimate conclusion can be drawn from these data.

Subclinical hypogonadism mediated by immunosupression [125], or decreased mitochondrial DNA content in oocytes from HIV1-infected HAART-treated females, may explain the poor results [127]. All in all, the number of available studies is limited, which makes it difficult to draw conclusions.

No consensus has been reached about miscarriage rates after IVF. Some authors have shown this rate increases [113], while other studies have observed that it falls in the same range as that of the general population [115, 126].

Table 2. Managing HIV-1-Infected Couples

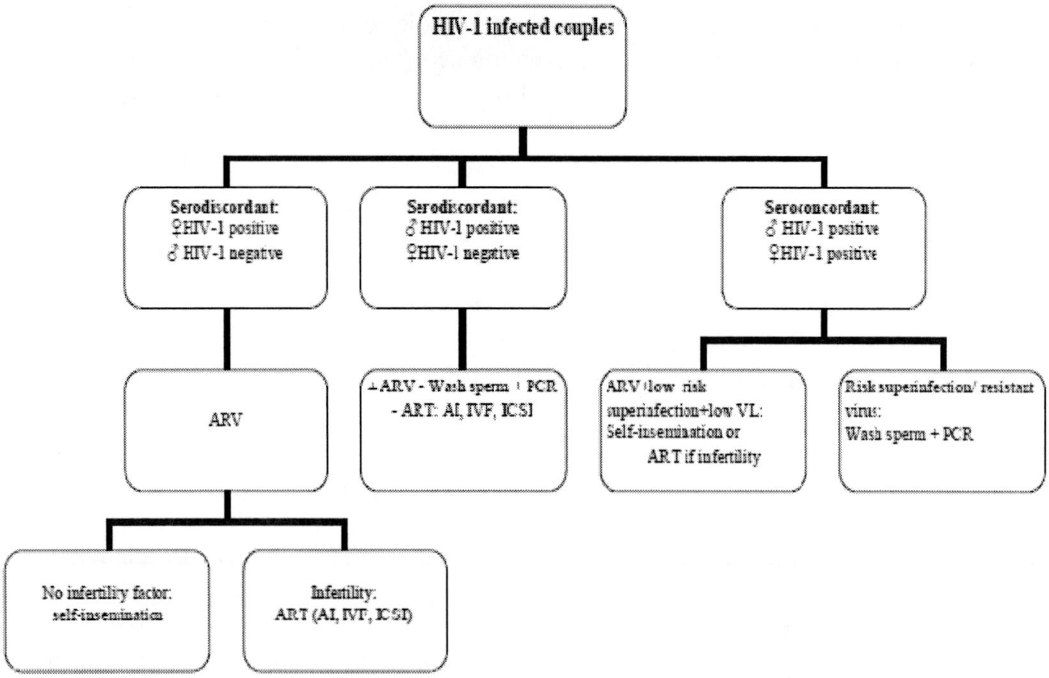

ARV: Antiretroviral. ART: Assisted reproduction techniques. AI: Artificial insemination. IVF: *In vitro* fertilization. ICSI: Intracytoplasmatic sperm injection.. Vl viral load.

Serodiscordant Couples: HIV-1 Positive Males

Natural conception outside the framework of effective HAART and with confirmed detectable viral load in plasma should be strongly discouraged.

Given the high cost involved in carrying out ART (after sperm washing), planned intercourse has been considered in cases of an HIV-1 infected male with undetectable plasma viremia undergoing HAART for > 6 months for 6-12 ovulations. Although HAART can reduce the semen viral load to an undetectable level in most patients [128, 129], the persistence of HIV RNA and/or infected cells in semen has been reported in up to 10% of men taking various antiretroviral treatment combinations, despite an undetectable blood viral load [130, 131]. The residual viral load detected in semen is generally low but appears to be extremely variable amongst individuals [131, 132].

Restriction of unprotected sexual intercourse until the woman's fertile days is necessary to minimise the risk [133]. Two studies have stated that serodiscordant couples in whom the infected partner had an undetectable blood viral load under prolonged HAART could safely have unprotected intercourses in the absence of other sexually transmitted infections (STIs) [134, 135].

In the literature, it appears that although drastically reduced, the possibility of transmitting HIV despite an undetectable blood viral load following HAART remains in a subset of patients, approximately 0.5 per 100 person-years [103]. This persistence of HIV excretion in the semen of a subset of individuals undergoing HAART has potentially important consequences for the transmission of the virus. The critical inoculum for sexual transmission is unknown [136].

So, it seems less cautious to abandon the recommendations of safe sex in serodiscordant couples desiring a child. The recourse to medically assisted procreation is advised, provided that evidence from further studies does not show that unprotected sexual intercourse, targeted to fertile days, has no unexpected harmful consequences [137].

Sperm Washing

Sperm washing aims to separate spermatozoa from all other semen components, and to thereby obtain an HIV-1-free spermatozoal fraction containing sufficient morphologically normal spermatozoa with progressive motility [139]. This process involves double gradient centrifugation followed by swim up because it is more effective when removing HIV-1 RNA than double gradient centrifugation alone.

As a control, an aliquot of washed sperm should be PCR-tested prior to using the sample for treatment. The risk of sample contamination, that is, of having detectable HIV-1 in sperm after washing, is 5-6% [140]. Sensitivity of testing varies, and the nested PCR that we carried out lowers the detection limits to 1 copy HIV-1 RNA/DNA [141]. Moreover, it is likely that this methodology is responsible for the post-washing positive rates of around 10% [114, 138], which is higher than the other values found in the literature; obviously, these other studies used tests with lower sensitivity.

HIV-1 viremia should be reduced in the infected partner by using ARV drugs prior to the fertility treatment because sperm washing appears more effective [114]. Nevertheless, our group observed no benefits in administering ARV before washing [142]. Nicopoullos et al showed in a recent review their experience after 10 years of sperm washing that there was no significant difference in any parameter between the samples in which viral load (VL) was detectable and in those where it was undetectable. The use of HAART significantly decreased the total sperm count, progressive motility, post-preparation count and TMCI (total motile count inseminated); a proportion of abnormal forms was also significantly increased and a significant negative correlation between the duration of HAART use and sample quality was also observed [139].

After semen processing, intrauterine insemination (IUI) is the first therapeutic alternative given the fact that a high percentage of couples are voluntarily infertile and do not have significant fertility issues. IVF or ICSI is recommended when the fertility study reveals an associated female factor or when seminal quality after washing is insufficient for IUI. (Table 2).

The average pregnancy rate in IUI in the literature is around 20% [60, 140, 143-152]. However, mechanisms to encourage the use of fresh sperm wherever possible, such as the use of GnRH antagonists, to delay ovulation may further improve cycle outcome [138]. In IVF/ICSI, the average pregnancy rate is 38% [8,121, 142, 151, 153-155].

IUI and IVF/ICSI results show that the reproductive efficacy of these techniques after sperm washing does not seem significantly affected. Accordingly, we have seen that HIV-1 infection in serodiscordant couples (SDCs) with an infected male does not appear to have a significantly negative impact on embryo development or ICSI outcome when compared with a tubal factor infertility control group [155].

In azoospermic HIV-positive males, an appropriate sperm count is difficult to achieve, especially in non obstructive azoospermia. In the first reported case, sperm was obtained by micro-epididymal aspiration, and the sample was frozen after density gradient preparation and tested for HIV-RNA and DNA; finally, ICSI was performed with frozen sperm [99]. Recently we published the first report of TESE (testicular sperm extraction) -ICSI in azoospermic seropositive males (VIH or hepatitis C) , and showed that it is a viable approach, and that such patients should be considered for HAART if these techniques, together with sperm washing and PCR confirmation of the viral absence, can be performed [156].

Couples should receive counselling to practice safe sex and to understand that it is necessary to use condoms through fertility treatment, in pregnancy and in the postpartum period.

In 2006, a case of HIV seroconversion in a women preparing for ICSI was described [156]. Should the condom accidentally break, it is recommended to postpone any HAART for six months for the purpose of covering window of risk infection [157].

Controls must be done throughout the whole pregnancy and the postpartum period to ensure that there is no sexual transmission of HIV, and even some groups recommend doing tests on the newborn baby. If pregnancy is not achieved after HAART, tests are also recommended [112]

Co-infected males with HIV-1 and hepatitis C undergoing assisted reproduction have similar viral loads and CD4 concentrations as those males infected only with HIV-1. IVF performance and outcomes are also similar in terms of fertilisation rates, numbers of normally cleaving embryos, and of embryo implantation and clinical pregnancy rates. However, morbidity among co-infected males is significantly higher [158].

Seroconcordant HIV-1-Positive Couples

There are different criteria for ART management given the risk of death for both partners, and of leaving children orphaned [13]. This issue should, at least, be discussed with the couple before starting ART.

A genotype HIV-1 study should be done to assess whether both partners are infected with the same viral subtype and if they receive antiretroviral treatment until a non-detectable viral load in blood has been achieved [2]. Semen processing is always advised when resistant virus is present, because HAART options could be limited if this virus is transmitted.

If both partners receive ARV with a viral load of < 50 copies/ml, and the female has a low risk of superinfection, the alternative would be to perform self-insemination [112], timed intercourse [2], or ART if infertility is present. Monthly monitoring of the male is recommended for the early detection of a resistant virus for cases in which only the male receives ARV and has a blood plasma HIV-1 of < 50 copies/ml, or if only the female receives ARV and has a viral load of < 50 copies/ml with no resistant virus detected in the male.

If neither partner receives ARV and there is no superinfection risk, the procedure will be the same as in the aforementioned case. If there is a risk of superinfection, sperm washing and PCR should be carried out, and the same attitude is advisable when only the female receives ARV and presents a viral load of < 50 copies/ml with a resistant virus detected in the male [120] (Table 2).

Hepatitis B Virus (HBV)

Two billion people are infected worldwide with hepatitis B virus (HBV), 360 million present chronic infections, and 600,000 die every year from HBV-related liver disease or hepatocellular carcinoma [160]. Chronic HBV infection develops in 2-6% of adults, 30-60% of young children, and as many as 90% of infants (<1 year) exposed to HBV [161]. Approximately 25% of regular sexual contacts of HBV-infected persons will become seropositive [162].

Outside high-risk collectives, like i.v. drug addicts and homosexuals, the virus especially spreads sexually or vertically with high level of contagiousness since it is present and infectious not only in blood, but also in semen, saliva and vaginal secretion.

The most serious health consequence of HBV infection occurs in those people who develop a chronic infection. A chronic HBV carrier is defined as an individual with HBsAg detectable in serum for more than 6 months. The carrier state occurs equally in both men and women, and carriers can transmit infection to others. HBeAg positivity is associated with a higher rate of transmitting infection in chronic HBsAg carriers.

Strict adherence to standard precautions and vaccination with the Hepatitis B vaccine is the most effective way of preventing HBV infection [163]. It may be administered to pregnant women and women contemplating pregnancy [161].

Screening for the HBs antigen is essential in all pregnant women because the active and passive immunoprophylaxis for the newborn will avoid the majority of possible infections if mothers are seropositive [164]. When the HBs antigen is found in pregnant women, a specialist should be consulted, and the family should undergo complete serologic testing (HBs antigen, anti-HBc and anti-HBs antibodies).

Hepatitis B in Females

Pregnancy seems to have no influence on HBV chronic infection, and vice versa [164]. Acute HBV occurs in one or two of every 1,000 pregnancies, of which 1.5% of pregnant women will be chronic HBV carriers. There is no evidence that HBV infection is more common in pregnancy.

The incidence of spontaneous abortion during the first trimester in patients with acute viral hepatitis is higher. Likewise, there is a higher incidence of preterm labour when viral hepatitis occurs during the third trimester. These higher incidences of spontaneous abortion and preterm delivery are probably no higher than those reported for other febrile illnesses [165].

Transmission may occur as a result of intrapartum exposure, transplacental transmission, and breast-feeding. Approximately 20%-30% of HBsAg seropositive patients transmit the virus to their newborns in the absence of an immunoprophylaxis. In women who are HBsAg-positive and HBeAg-positive, the frequency of transmission increases to 90% [166,167] (Table 1).

Although a high level of HBV viremia may imply higher incidence of materno-foetal transmission, the magnitude of the increased risk and the exact level of viremia at which the risk becomes significant remain unknown. Thus, viral DNA levels must be monitored and conception must be attempted when the viral load is low. HBV infection has been detected in newborns and abortions of HBV seronegative mothers. Since HBV DNA has been detected in semen and spermatozoa, a possible father-neonate transmission of HBV has been inferred [168,169]. Indeed, HBV vertical transmission from father to foetus was consequently confirmed by direct sequencing [168]. More studies should concentrate on the detection of the HBV genome in gametes and embryos.

The frequency of transmission also depends on the time at which infection occurs during pregnancy. If acute maternal infection occurs in the first trimester, up to 10% of infants will be HbsAg-positive, yet if it appears during the third trimester, 90% of neonates without a prophylaxis will be positive (Table 1).

Infants born to HBsAg-positive mothers should receive both Hepatitis B immune globulin (HBIG) and the Hepatitis B vaccine within 12 hours of birth, followed by two more HBV vaccine injections in the first 6 months of life [170]. The combined use of passive (HBIG) and active immunisation is 85% to 95% effective in preventing neonatal HBV infection [161].

The causes of immunisation failure are unclear, although high levels of maternal viremia [171] and intrauterine infection [172] probably contribute. Indeed they were recently attributed to HBV strains with mutations in the surface protein (HBsAg) [173].

Despite this prophylaxis being highly effective, women with very high viral loads may receive lamivudine treatment at the end of pregnancy to lower the viral load and, therefore, the risk of chronic carriage in the child. Nevertheless, the role of this drug in this situation is still to be clearly defined [164].

Vaccination is recommended for the non-infected partner in serodiscordant couples [161]. Vaccines can be safely administered during pregnancy (3 doses are better than 2) to non-HVB infected pregnant women because they provide the foetus with passive immunity by transferring antibodies [174-176].

Currently, no information is available about how HBV affects the reproductive function in female carriers. HBVDNA has been detected in the ovum at different stages such as HBcAg and in granular cells and interstitial cells of the ovary. HBV DNA is distributed mainly in the nucleus, but can also be detected in the cytoplasm, and it may be an important mechanism of HBV vertical transmission [177].

Another aspect to consider is the tubal disease, which is present in 45.5% of infected women [178], owing to the sexual transmission common to both conditions. However, the prevalence of the HBV carrier status among infertile women is comparable to that in the general obstetric population. This observation suggests that chronic HBV infection is unlikely to be a significant cause of infertility, even in a hyperendemic area [169].

Hepatitis B in Males

The presence of HBV in different testicle cell types and ejaculated semen samples has been proved in chronically infected males [179,180].

Sperm concentration, viability and normal morphology were significantly lower in HBV-seropositive men than in the controls [181]. Lee et al also showed a reduction in the percentage of normal sperm morphology in HBV-seropositive husbands compared with seronegative counterparts in IVF cycles [182].

Assisted Reproductive Techniques

Serodiscordant Couples: HBV-Positive Females

It is advisable to vaccinate males, as is the use of condoms for their own protection until immunity is achieved (anti-HBs titres >10 IU/l) [161]. If males do not achieved immunity after vaccination and seroconversion is absent after revaccination, then intrauterine insemination should be consider to decrease the risk of transmission [161].

From a reproductive viewpoint, assisted reproduction treatments will only be carried out if the female presents the following conditions: acute infection has successfully remitted, no severe liver disease, HVBeAg is negative, and a low viral load (probably of < 10^6 copies/ml).

From this point onwards, the options to achieve pregnancy should be ART as indicated for each case, and in accordance with the exact sterility problem (Table 3).

There has been controversy about the effect of hepatitis B virus (HBV) infection on pregnancy outcome after IVF treatment. Pirwany described a reduced pregnancy rate (PR) in HBV-infected women [183], while others showed no significant differences [182] or obtained only significantly higher PRs and implantation rates [169].

Since HBV can be found in cervical and vaginal secretions, Lam et al speculated that HBV infection may induce inflammatory changes in the female lower genital tract, and that IVF and embryo transfer treatment can overcome some of these inhibitory effects [169].

Serodiscordant Couples: HBV Positive Males

In chronic seropositive males, it is advisable to vaccinate the female partner and to use condoms until immunological protection has been achieved in the female partner. Once immunity has been achieved, the couple will be able to attempt to conceive through the ART indicated for their specific sterility problem (Table 3).

Table 3. Managing Couples Infected with HBV

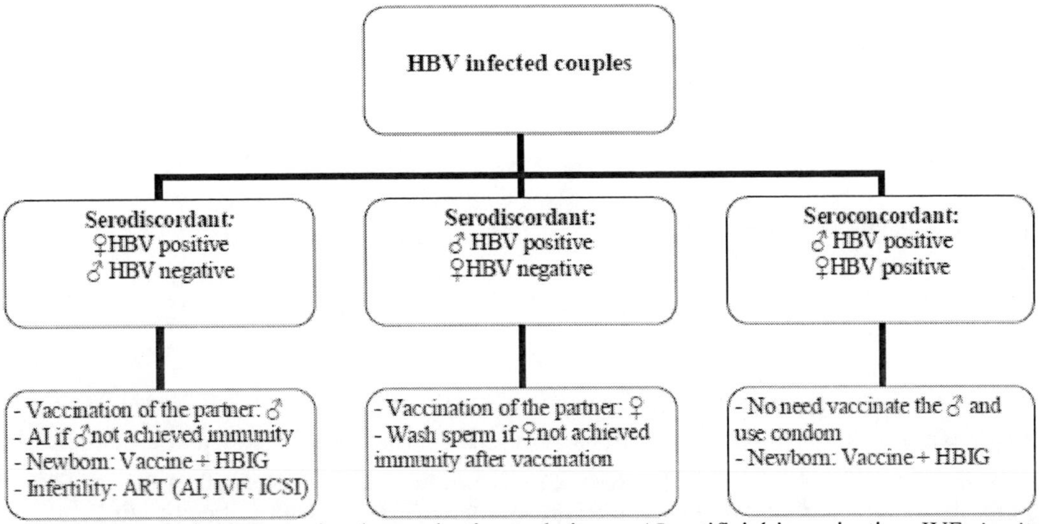

ARV: Antiretroviral. ART: Assisted reproduction techniques. AI: artificial insemination. IVF: *in vitro* fertilization. ICSI: intracytoplasmatic sperm injection. VL: Viral load. HBIG Immunoglobulin against hepatitis B.

In this way, risk of transmission to the female and offspring will be avoided or minimised. Only the sperm washing technique will be carried out to reduce the viral load of HBV in this fluid when the female partner has not achieved immunity after precise vaccination. After the sperm procedure, and once the absence of the virus has been verified *via* PCR, semen will be used for self-inseminations, artificial insemination or *in vitro* fertilisation in accordance with the couple's characteristics.

The IVF results available in HBV-positive men show no differences with the control group in terms of seminal parameters or implantation and pregnancy rates [169,182,183]

Seroconcordant HVB-Positive Couples

The same advise used when the female partner is seropositive applies when both partners are HBV seropositive; however neither vaccination nor condom use is necessary.

Hepatitis C Virus (HCV)

Hepatitis C affects > 1% of the world population and is the most frequent cause of chronic viral hepatitis since 80% will develop chronic liver disease [162]. Co-infection with HIV-1 or HBV is associated with an increased risk of developing cirrhosis or hepatocellular carcinoma.

HCV is a blood-borne virus transmitted through percutaneous exposures to blood (e.g., transfusions or transplants), needle sticks or the contamination of supplies shared among hemodialysis patients or IV drug users. HCV RNA has also been detected in saliva, breast milk, urine, menstrual fluid and semen. Therefore, sexual and vertical transmission has been suggested to be alternative HCV transmission modes.

Currently, combination therapy using interferon alpha plus ribavirin provides a better response rate compared with monotherapy, and is now considered the first-line therapy [184]. Although both drugs are contraindicated during pregnancy, interferon use in early pregnancy has shown no teratogenic effects. Lack of teratogenicity is believed to be due to the simple fact that this drug does not pass through the placenta. Ribavirin should not be used by pregnant women, women attempting pregnancy, or male partners trying to conceive [184]. Similarly, mothers taking antiviral medication should not breast-feed owing to the possibility of adverse reactions for their infants.

Hepatitis C in Females

The risk of sexual transmission for women is higher than it is for men. However, it is low if compared with other viral infections. For HCV-discordant, monogamous couples, the seroconversion rate after ten years is 2.5%. This risk of transmission increases in cases of genital lesion given traumatic intercourse or associated sexually transmitted diseases.

The timing and route of vertical transmission remain unclear and it is not known whether transmission is transplacental or takes place during delivery. Nonetheless, there are reports in which at least one third and as much as half the infected children acquired infection in the uterus. The seroprevalence of hepatitis C among United States prenatal populations is 2.3-4.5%, and is as high as 33% when mothers have HIV-1 co-infection [161].

A correlation between the risk of vertical transmission and maternal viral burden has been described. This risk of transmission for females with antibodies against HCV and negative HCV RNA is less than 1-3%, and over 4-10% if it is positive [185]. A titer from which vertical transmission occurs has not been established [186], although no women whose titer was below 10^4 copies/mL transmitted the virus to their infants. Likewise, the close association between vertical HCV transmission and maternal viral titers over 10^6 copies/mL has been confirmed in HIV-negative mothers, reaching up to 36% [187]. (Table 1).

Recent data indicate that perinatal HCV transmission is greater in women co-infected with HIV, ranging from 10% to 15% [117, 188]. According to these results, it has been postulated that HIV-infected women who transmitted HCV more frequently presented higher maternal HCV viremia. Unfortunately, there is no prospective study available on HCV-infected females with HIV seropositivity and HIV seronegativity to test this hypothesis definitively.

Viral heterogeneity of HCV is also an additional risk factor for vertical transmission. Despite the few studies available that have centred on the role of HCV genotypes as a risk factor, HCV genotypes 1b and 3a seem to be most commonly transmitted [188]. In another study, infants infected with genotype 1 were significantly more likely to present evidence of intrauterine infection than those derived from other genotypes [189].

Among the maternal risk factors that may increase transmission, history of drug use, irrespectively of HIV infection, is worth mentioning [190]. One explanation for this is that drug use is believed to impair the immune system function and to induce tolerance to viral infections.

On the other hand, pregnancy (in the absence of cirrhosis and portal hypertension) does not induce deteriorated liver function. As regards the adverse effects of the obstetrical results, none appears to have increased. Yet Pergam et al found that infants of HCV-positive mothers were more likely to present low birth weight, small-for-gestational age, require assisted ventilation and have to be admitted to a neonatal intensive care unit (NICU) [191]. The newborn has high levels of alanine aminotransferase (ALT) and anti-VHC antibodies, which gradually decrease in non-infected children and more slowly in those whose mothers had viremia.

Hepatitis C in Males

HCV can be found in the semen of seropositive males at a rate of between 5% and 30% [192]. It is, however, necessary to examine this information very carefully as PCR inhibitors are present in ejaculated fluid. Therefore, the presence of the virus in semen can be associated with male sterility through an immunity or inflammatory reaction, or via a direct toxic effect [193].

There is a low, yet measurable, risk of sexual transmission via semen [161]. When the male partner is HCV-infected, sperm washing can reduce the viral load in semen and is a recommended measure to reduce the risk of transmission to partners [181].

As with hepatitis B, sperm concentration, viability and normal morphology were significantly lower in HCV-seropositive men than in controls, and sperm concentration after sperm washing was also significantly higher in controls than in HCV patients [181].

Assisted Reproductive Techniques

Serodiscordant Couples: HCV-Positive Females

Despite there being controversy on this point, the American Fertility Society (AFS) [114] and the Control Diseases Centre (CDC) [4] consider hepatitis C a sexually transmitted disease and advise the use of condoms to lower the risk of transmission to partners when attempting to conceive. However, Thome et al analysed 80 qualifying reports of heterosexual transmission of HC, concluding that the weight of evidence shows there is no increased risk of sexual transmission of HCV among heterosexual couples in regular relationships. This risk increases among persons with multiple sexual partners. There appears to be a real increased risk for women co-infected with human immunodeficiency virus (HIV) or with other sexually transmitted infections [194].

Although shedding HCV RNA in the female genital tract is associated with detection of haemoglobin (even if menstruation does not occur), HCV RNA was not detected in cervicovaginal fluids in post-hysterectomy women on any day regardless of whether haemoglobin was detected, so it seems that the presence of cervix is necessary. Clinicians should consider advising premenopausal women who are concerned about transmitting infection that infectivity may increase during menstruation [195].

From the reproductive viewpoint, assisted reproduction treatments should be carried out only in cases in which acute infection has disappeared, in the absence of severe liver disease and HIV co-infection, and when the viral load (DNA) is $< 1x\ 10^6$ copies/ml (375.000 UI/ml) [114]. Following these inclusion criteria, the risk of vertical transmission is minimised.

Unprotected sexual relations are only advisable during either natural or induced ovulation to attempt pregnancy when the possible risk of transmission is known (5%) [196]. The use of condoms is advisable for seropositive females and seronegative males when pregnancy is not desired. In our opinion, it is advisable to perform self-inseminations instead of unprotected sexual relations when no obvious infertility factor is found. The options to achieve pregnancy include insemination or the ART indicated for each case in accordance with the sterility problem (Table **4**). These recommendations probably should be evaluated again in light of the results shown recently in the review by Thome et al [194].

HCV infection may affect the results of an assisted reproduction cycle. Englert et al recently published a retrospective study which demonstrated a statistically significant association between HCV infection in women and altered ovarian function: cancelled cycles increase, while lower oestradiol levels are achieved and fewer oocytes are obtained for increased stimulation in non-cancelled cycles [197].

Serodiscordant Couples: HCV-Positive Males

The sexual transmission risk, together with publications proving the possibility of cross-contamination between patients during assisted reproductive techniques [185,198], mean it is advisable to submit semen for selection by centrifugation followed by the swim-up technique. Motile spermatozoa are divided into two parts, of which one is frozen and the other is used to detect HCV RNA. If negative, the frozen, safe, non-infected cryopreserved semen fraction should be used for assisted reproduction [142] (Table 4), although this attitude may be questionable given the recent data reported by Thome et al [194].

Low implantation rates for HCV-seropositive males [22] and low fertilisation rates when compared with HIV-positive males, or those co-infected by HCV, have been described; however, there are no significant differences in pregnancy rates [142]. Nonetheless in a retrospective case-controlled, university-based study, Prisant et al observed that the clinical pregnancy rate for HIV-1 or HCV male carriers in fertile serodiscordant couples did not significantly differ from that for seronegative controls [199].

Recently, we published the first report of pregnancy after TESE (testicular sperm extraction)-ICSI in azoospermic seropositive HCV males together with sperm washing and PCR confirmation of the viral absence [156].

Treatment with peginterferon-alpha and ribavirin should be considered prior to fertility treatment to lower the viral load [200]; however as in the case of HIV, our group does not consider it necessary [142]. The reason for our posture is the evidence available indicating no relationship between the blood viral load and the semen viral load [201]. Thus, the viral load in blood is uninformative and there is no need to eliminate the virus to perform assisted reproduction [202].

When semen samples are collected, use of ribavirin is not advisable as it can have adverse effects on germinal cells [203]. As this drug is believed to cause new mutations, two contraception forms are recommended for avoiding pregnancy during therapy: pregnancy testing performed monthly and delaying pregnancy for 6 months after discontinuing therapy in either partner.

Table 4. Managing HCV-infected Couples

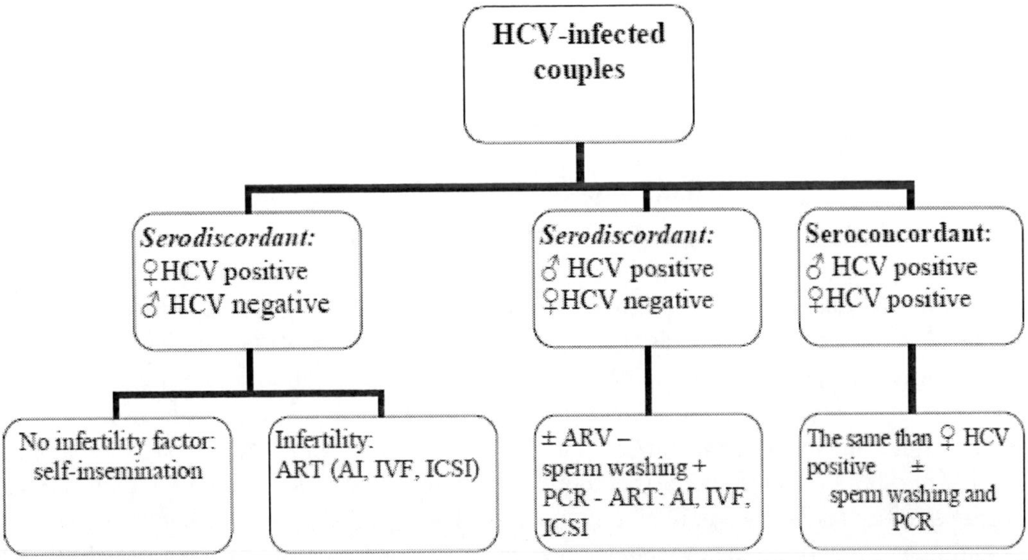

ARV: Antiretroviral. ART: Assisted reproduction techniques. AI: artificial insemination. IVF: in vitro fertilisation. ICSI: intracytoplasmatic sperm injection. VL: Viral load.

Seroconcordant Hcv-Positive Couples

When both partners are seropositive, the same as when the female is seropositive, it would be advisable to use sperm washing followed by PCR to avoid the transmission of different viral genotypes (in case we are not certain that they are the same).

Laboratory Recommendations

Health professionals who care for patients with chronic viral diseases are exposed to semen, blood or follicular fluid that are potentially infected with HIV, HCV or HBV [21, 204, 205]. Although the main risk lies in needle prickings or splash injuries, it is minimised if standard universal precautions to prevent infectious disease transmission are taken [14].

Safety guidelines include the following: 1) handle all body fluids as though they were contaminated, 2) wear protective non-toxic gloves, glasses or goggles, mouth mask or full face protection if formation of aerosols or droplets is involved, 3) cap tubes while centrifuging and close the centrifuge when in use, 4) clean and decontaminate bench tops and instruments regularly, 5) use mechanical pipetting devices, 6) provide a hand-washing sink and an eyewash station, 7) wash hands after removing gowns and gloves, and immediately if they become contaminated, 8) ban eating, drinking, smoking, application of make-up, or manipulation of contact lenses in the laboratory, 9) do not store food and beverages in refrigerators used to store clinical specimens and other laboratory material, 10) implement a bio-hazardous materials disposal plan and 11) vaccinate employees against HBV [1].

In addition, some special safety procedures have been developed to reduce professional or cross-contamination risks between staff and patients since the IVF laboratory is a good place to promote cell survival, thus the development and growth of viruses and bacteria. Therefore, working surfaces and equipment should be cleaned with additional disinfecting agents; infected patients should be treated in an isolated manner, leaving enough time for decontamination; oocytes and embryos must be placed in incubators with separate specific compartments.

Samples from these patients must be handled in a separate high-security technically-adapted laboratory or laboratory area to ensure minimal cross-contamination risks to uninfected gametes and embryos [206]. Laboratories working with infected patients must have an airtight chamber, a vertical laminar chamber for viral cultures with 100% recirculated filtered air, safety access procedures and a separate area to treat biological liquids [112].

For several years, there has been much discussion about the potential for cross-contamination in liquid nitrogen storage tanks. Cross-contamination is the transmission of a pathogen from a cryopreserved gamete/embryo to another during storage in liquid nitrogen which results in the production of disease in the offspring from that contaminated gamete/embryo. To date, there is no published report of cross-contamination between reproductive tissues in cryogenic storage under IVF laboratory working conditions, although there are many reports of the procedures occurring before screening for pathogens [207,208]. There are some reports of contamination under entirely unrelated conditions (e.g., blood banking) [209] or contrived scenarios that bear no relation to embryo culture or embryo cryopreservation conditions [210].

Samples must be allocated to separate storage devices to avoid mixed infected specimens with general specimens [211], and high-security straws should be used instead of breakable ones [212]. High-security straws are highly effective in human embryo cryopreservation because they provide higher cryosurvival and implantation rates, as well as a lower risk of cross-contamination compared to conventional straws [213]. Thermal sealing of straws is most recommended, as is disinfecting the outer sample container surfaces before freezing and after thawing to reduce the risk of contamination [207]. Vapour phase of liquid nitrogen (VPLN2) as an alternative to liquid nitrogen (LN2) is another proposed, safer storage method [214].

Before introducing new techniques into cryopreservation (e.g., decontaminants) which might prove suitable for other tissue types or other species, proper testing must be done to avoid embryonic death, lower pregnancy rates (PR) and possible increased mutagenesis.

References

[1] Steyaert SR, Leroux-Roels GG, Dhont M. Infections in IVF: review and guidelines. *Hum. Reprod. Update* 2000; 6: 432-41.

[2] Williams CD, Finnerty JJ, Newberry YG, *et al.* Reproduction in couples who are affected by human immunodeficiency virus: medical, ethical, and legal considerations. *Am. J. Obstet .Gynecol.* 2003; 189: 333-41.

[3] Lesourd F, Izopet J, Mervan C, *et al.* Transmissions of hepatitis C virus during the ancillary procedures for assisted conception. *Hum. Reprod.* 2000; 15: 1083-5.

[4] Centres for Disease Control and Prevention (CDC). Sexually transmitted diseases treatment guidelines, 2006. *MMWR Recomm. Rep.* 2006; 55: 1-94.

[5] Van den Eede. Investigation and treatment of infertile couples: ESHRE guidelines for good clinical and laboratory practice. European Society of Human Reproduction and Embryology. *Hum. Reprod.* 1995; 10: 1246-71.

[6] Sherr L, Barry N. Fatherhood and HIV-positive heterosexual men. *HIV Med.* 2004; 5: 258-63.

[7] Paiva V, Filipe EV, Santos N, *et al.* The right to love: the desire for parenthood among men living with HIV. *Reprod. Health Matters* 2003; 11: 91-100.

[8] Sauer MV, Chang PL. Establishing a clinical program for human immunodeficiency virus 1-seropositive men to father seronegative children by means of *in vitro* fertilization with intracytoplasmic sperm injection. *Am. J. Obstet. Gynecol.* 2002; 187: 1121.

[9] Ohl J, Partisani M. The desire to become a parent when infected with human immunodeficiency virus, hepatitis C virus or hepatitis B virus. *Gynecol. Obstet. Fertil.* 2007; 35: 1035-8.

[10] Sauer MV. American physicians remain slow to embrace the reproductive needs of human immunodeficiency virus-infected patients. *Fertil. Steril.* 2006; 85: 295-7.

[11] Thornton AC, Romanelli F, Collins JD. Reproduction decision making for couples affected by HIV: a review of the literatura. *Top HIV Med.* 2004; 12: 61-7.

[12] FIGO Committee for the Ethical Aspects of Human Reproduction nd Women´s Health. *Int. J. Gynecol. Obstet.* 2006; 93: 187-8.

[13] Shenfield F, Pennings G, Cohen J, *et al.* C; ESHRE Ethics and Law Task Force. Task Force 8: ethics of medically assisted fertility treatment for HIV positive men and women. *Hum. Reprod.* 2004; 19: 2454-6.

[14] Ethics Committee of the American Society for Reproductive Medicine. Human immunodeficiency virus and infertility treatment. *Fertil. Steril.* 2002; 77: 212-22.

[15] Zutlevics T. Should ART be offered to HIV-serodiscordant and HIV-seroconcordant couples: an ethical discussion? *Hum. Reprod.* 2006; 21: 1956-60.

[16] Gilling-Smith C, Smith JR, Semprini AE. HIV and infertility: time to treat. There's no justification for denying treatment to parents who are HIV positive. *BMJ* 2001; 322: 566-7.

[17] Minkoff H, Santoro N. Ethical considerations in the treatment of infertility in women with human immunodeficiency virus infection. *N. Engl. J. Med.* 2000; 342: 1748-50.

[18] Minkoff H. Human immunodeficiency virus and infertility services: the glass is half full. *Fertil. Steril.* 2006; 85: 290-2.

[19] American College of Obstetrics and Gynecology. ACOG Committee Opinion No. 389, December 2007. Human immunodeficiency virus. *Obstet. Gynecol.* 2007; 110: 1473-8.

[20] Daar ES, Daar JF. Human immunodeficiency virus and fertility care: embarking on a path of knowledge and access. *Fertil. Steril.* 2006; 85: 298-300.

[21] Gilling-Smith C, Nicopoullos JD, Semprini AE, Frodsham LC. HIV and reproductive care--a review of current practice. *BJOG* 2006; 113: 869-78.

[22] Englert Y, Lesage B, Van Vooren JP, *et al.* Medically assisted reproduction in the presence of chronic viral diseases. *Hum. Reprod. Update* 2004;10:149-62.

[23] UNAIDS - Joint United Nations Programme on HIV/AIDS. New report on global AIDS epidemic (December2009). www.unaids.org/ en/HIV_data/2007GlobalReport/default.asp.

[24] Shors AR. The global epidemiology of HIV/AIDS. *Dermatol. Clin.* 2006; 24: 413-20.

[25] Bokazhanova A, Rutherford GW. The epidemiology of HIV and AIDS in the world. *Coll. Antropol.* 2006; 30 (Suppl 2): 3-10.

[26] Mostad SB, Kreiss JK. Shedding of HIV-1 in the genital tract. *AIDS* 1996; 10: 1305-15.

[27] Clemetson DB, Moss GB, Willerford DM, *et al.* Detection of HIV DNA in cervical and vaginal secretions. Prevalence and correlates among women in Nairobi, Kenya. *JAMA* 1993; 269: 2860-4.

[28] Money DM, Arikan YY, Remple V, *et al.* Genital tract and plasma human immunodeficiency virus viral load throughout the menstrual cycle in women who are infected with ovulatory human immunodeficiency virus. *Am. J. Obstet. Gynecol.* 2003; 188: 122-8.

[29] Kovacs A, Wasserman SS, Burns D, *et al.* Determinants of HIV-1 shedding in the genital tract of women. *Lancet* 2001; 358: 1593- 601.

[30] Coombs RW, Wright DJ, Reichelderfer PS, *et al.* Variation of human immunodeficiency virus type 1 viral RNA levels in the female genital tract: implications for applying measurements to individual women. *J. Infect. Dis.* 2001; 184: 1187-91.

[31] Mostad SB, Jackson S, Overbaugh J, *et al.* Cervical and vaginal shedding of human immunodeficiency virus type 1-infected cells throughout the menstrual cycle. *J. Infect. Dis.* 1998; 178: 983-91.

[32] Villanueva JM, Ellerbrock TV, Lennox JL, *et al.* The menstrual cycle does not affect human immunodeficiency virus type 1 levels in vaginal secretions. *J. Infect. Dis.* 2002; 185: 170-7.

[33] Mostad SB, Overbaugh J, DeVange DM, *et al.* Hormonal contraception, vitamin A deficiency, and other risk factors for shedding of HIV-1 infected cells from the cervix and vagina. *Lancet* 1997; 350: 922-7.

[34] Hinz S, McCormack D, vander Spuy ZM. Endocrine function in HIV-infected women. *Gynecol. Endocrinol.* 2002; 16: 33-38.

[35] Chirgwin KD, Feldman J, Muneyyirci-Delale O, Landesman S, Minkoff H. Menstrual function in human immunodeficiency virusinfected women without acquired immunodeficiency syndrome. *J. Acquir. Immune Defic. Syndr. Hum. Retrovirol.* 1996; 12: 489-94.

[36] Clark RA, Mulligan K, Stamenovic E, *et al.* Frequency of anovulation and early menopause among women enrolled in selected adult AIDS clinical trials group studies. *J. Infect. Dis.* 2001; 184: 1325-7.

[37] Ohl J, Partisani M, Demangeat C, Binder-Foucard F, Nisand I, et al. Alterations of ovarian reserve tests in Human Immunodeficiency Virus (HIV)-infected women]. *Gynecol. Obstet. Fertil.* 2010 May;38(5):313-7.

[38] Blair JM, Hanson DL, Jones JL, Dworkin MS. Trends in pregnancy rates among women with human immunodeficiency virus. *Obstet. Gynecol.* 2004; 103: 663-8.

[39] Santoro N, Arnsten JH, Buono D, Howard AA, Schoenbaum EE. Impact of street drug use, HIV infection, and highly active antiretroviral therapy on reproductive hormones in middle-aged women. *J. Womens Health (Larchmt).* 2005 Dec;14(10):898-905.

[40] Sellmeyer DE, Grunfeld C. Endocrine and metabolic disturbances in human immunodeficiency virus infection and the acquired immune deficiency syndrome. *Endocr. Rev.* 1996; 17(5): 518-32.

[41] Barbaro G. HIV infection, antiretroviral therapy and cardiovascular risk. *J. Cardiovasc. Risk* 2002; 9: 295-300.

[42] Santoro N, Lo Y, Moskaleva G, Arnsten JH, Floris-Moore M, et al. Factors affecting reproductive hormones in HIV-infected, substance-using middle-aged women. *Menopause.* 2007 Sep-Oct;14(5):859-65.

[43] Frankel RE, Selwyn PA, Mezger J, Andrews S. High prevalence of gynecologic disease among hospitalized women with human immunodeficiency virus infection. *Clin. Infect. Dis.* 1997; 25: 706- 12.

[44] Adesiyun AG, Ameh CA, Eka A. Hysterosalpingographic tubal abnormalities and HIV infection among black women with tubal infertility in sub-Saharan Africa. *Ecol. Obstet. Invest.* 2008; 66: 119- 22.

[45] Englert Y, Lesage B, Van Vooren JP, *et al.* Medically assisted reproduction in the presence of chronic viral diseases. *Hum. Reprod. Update* 2004; 10: 149-62.

[46] Clark RA, Mulligan K, Stamenovic E, *et al.* Frequency of anovulation and early menopause among women enrolled in selected adult AIDS clinical trials group studies. *J. Infect. Dis.* 2001; 184: 1325-7.

[47] Seifer DB, Golub ET, Lambert-Messerlian G, *et al.* Biologic markers of ovarian reserve and reproductive aging: application in a cohort study of HIV infection in women. *Fertil. Steril.* 2007; 88: 1645-52.

[48] Gregson S, Zaba B, Garnett GP. Low fertility in women with HIV and the impact of the epidemic on orphanhood and early childhood mortality in sub-Saharan Africa. *AIDS* 1999; 13: 249-57.
[49] Lo JC, Schambelan M. Reproductive function in human immunodeficiency virus infection. *J. Clin. Endocrinol Metab.* 2001; 86: 2338-43.
[50] Fiore S, Heard I, Thorne C, *et al.* Reproductive experience of HIVinfected women living in Europe. *Hum. Reprod.* 2008; 23: 2140-4.
[51] Kanniappan S, Jeyapaul MJ, Kalyanwala S. Desire for motherhood: exploring HIV-positive women's desires, intentions and decisionmaking in attaining motherhood. *AIDS Care* 2008; 20: 625-30.
[52] Gray GE, McIntyre JA. Effect of HIV on women. *AIDS Read* 2006; 16: 365-8, 373-7.
[53] Myer L, Carter RJ, Katyal M, Toro P, El-Sadr WM, et al. Impact of antiretroviral therapy on incidence of pregnancy among HIV-infected women in Sub-Saharan Africa: a cohort study. *PLoS Med.* 2010 Feb 9;7(2):e1000229.
[54] Sturt AS, Dokubo EK, Sint TT Antiretroviral therapy (ART) for treating HIV infection in ART-eligible pregnant women. *Cochrane Database of Systematic Reviews* 2010, Issue 3. Art. No.: CD008440
[55] Viganò A, Manzoni P, Riva S, *et al.* Hyperinsulinemia induced by highly active antiretroviral therapy in an adolescent with polycystic ovary syndrome who was infected with human immunodeficiency virus. *Fertil. Steril.* 2003; 79: 422-3.
[56] Johnsen S, Dolan SE, Fitch KV, *et al.* Absence of polycystic ovary syndrome features in human immunodeficiency virus-infected women despite significant hyperinsulinemia and truncal adiposity. *J. Clin. Endocrinol. Metab.* 2005; 90: 5596-604.
[57] Chouquet C, Richardson S, Burgard M, *et a*l. Timing of human immunodeficiency virus type 1 (HIV-1) transmission from mother to child: bayesian estimation using a mixture. *Stat. Med.* 1999; 18: 815-33.
[58] Kourtis AP, Lee FK, Abrams EJ, Jamieson DJ, Bulterys M. Mother-to-child transmission of HIV-1: timing and implications for prevention. *Lancet Infect. Dis.* 2006; 6: 726-32.
[59] Newell ML. Current issues in the prevention of mother-to-child transmission of HIV-1 infection. *Trans R Soc. Trop Med. Hyg.* 2006; 100: 1-5.
[60] European Collaborative Study. Mother - to - child transmission of HIV infection in the era of high active antiretroviral therapy. *Clin. Infect. Dis.* 2005; 40: 458-65.
[61] Panel on Treatment of HIV-Infected Pregnant Women and Prevention of Perinatal Transmission. Recommendations for Use of Antiretroviral Drugs in Pregnant HIV-1-Infected Women for Maternal Health and Interventions to Reduce Perinatal HIV Transmission in the United States. May 24, 2010; pp 1-117. http://aidsinfo.nih.gov/ContentFiles/PerinatalGL.pdf.
[62] Bessinger R, Clark R, Kissinger P, *et al.* Pregnancy is not associated with the progression of HIV disease in women attending an HIV outpatient program. *Am. J. Epidemiol.* 1998; 147: 434-40.
[63] Ahdieh L. Pregnancy and infection with human immunodeficiency virus. *Clin. Obstet. Gynecol.* 2001; 44: 154-66.
[64] French R, Brocklehurst P. The effect of pregnancy on survival in women infected with HIV: a systematic review of the literature and meta-analysis. *Br. J. Obstet. Gynaecol.* 1998; 105: 827-35.

[65] Tai JH, Udoji MA, Barkanic G, Byrne DW, Rebeiro PF, et al. Pregnancy and HIV disease progression during the era of highly active antiretroviral therapy. *J. Infect. Dis.* 2007 Oct 1;196(7):1044-52.

[66] Borzy MS, Connell RS, Kiessling AA. Detection of human immunodeficiency virus in cell-free seminal fluid. *J. Acquir. Immune Defic. Syndr.* 1988; 1: 419-24.

[67] Bagasra O, Farzadegan H, Seshamma T, *et al.* Detection of HIV-1 proviral DNA in sperm from HIV-1-infected men. *AIDS* 1994; 8:1669-74.

[68] Scofield VL, Rao B, Broder S, *et al.* HIV interaction with sperm. *AIDS* 1994; 8: 1733-6.

[69] Muciaccia B, Filippini A, Ziparo E, *et al.* Testicular germ cells of HIV-seropositive asymptomatic men are infected by the virus. *J. Reprod. Immunol.* 1998; 41: 81-93.

[70] Quayle AJ, Xu C, Mayer KH, *et al.* T lymphocytes and macrophages, but not motile spermatozoa, are a significant source of human immunodeficiency virus in semen. *J. Infect. Dis.* 1997; 176: 960-8.

[71] Pudney J, Nguyen H, Xu C, Anderson DJ. Microscopic evidence against HIV-1 infection of germ cells or attachment to sperm. *J. Reprod. Inmunol.* 1999; 44: 57-77.

[72] Anderson DJ, Politch JA, Martinez A, *et al.* White blood cells and HIV-1 in semen from vasectomised seropositive men. *Lancet* 1991; 338: 573-4.

[73] Cardona-Maya W, Velilla P, Montoya CJ, Cadavid A, Rugeles MT. Presence of HIV-1 DNA in spermatozoa from HIV-positive patients: changes in the semen parameters. *Curr. HIV Res.* 2009 Jul;7(4):418-24.

[74] Paranjpe S, Craigo J, Patterson B, *et al.* Subcompartmentalization of HIV-1 quasispecies between seminal cells and seminal plasma indicates their origin in distinct genital tissues. *AIDS Res. Hum. Retroviruses* 2002; 18: 1271-80.

[75] Le Tortorec A, Dejucq-Rainsford N. The male genital tract: A host for HIV. *Gynecol. Obstet. Fertil.* 2007; 35: 1245-50.

[76] Christeff N, Melchior JC, Mammes O, Gherbi N, Dalle MT, Nunez EA. Correlation between increased cortisol:DHEA ratio and malnutrition in HIV-positive men. *Nutrition* 1999; 15: 534-9.

[77] Collazos J, Martinez E, Mayo J, Ibarra S. Sexual hormones in HIVinfected patients: the influence of antiretroviral therapy. *AIDS* 2002; 16: 934-7.

[78] Collazos J. Sexual dysfunction in the highly active antiretroviral therapy era. *AIDS Rev.* 2007 Oct-Dec;9(4):237-45.

[79] Lowe SH. Is the male genital tract really a sanctuary site for HIV? Arguments that it is not. *AIDS* 2004; 18: 1353-62.

[80] Muller CH, Coombs RW, Krieger JN. Effects of clinical stage and immunological status on semen analysis results in human immunodeficiency virus type 1-seropositive men. *Andrologia* 1998; 30 (Suppl 1): 15-22.

[81] van Leeuwen E, Wit FW, Prins JM, Reiss P, van der Veen F, Repping S. Semen quality remains stable during 96 weeks of untreated human immunodeficiency virus-1 infection. *Fertil. Steril.* 2008; 90: 636-41.

[82] Sergerie M, Martinet S, Kiffer N, Teule R, Pasquier C, Bujan L. Impact des inhibiteurs nucléosidiques de la transcriptase inverse sur l'ADN mitochondrial et génomique des spermatozoïdes lors de l'Assistance Médicale à la Procréation. *Gynecologie Obstetrique and Fertilite.* 2004;32:841–849.

[83] Ball JK, Rowe T, Curran R, *et al.* Poor reduction of HIV-1 RNA titres in nucleoside reverse transcriptase inhibitor experienced patients treated with indinavir combination therapy. *Sex Transm. Infect.* 1999; 75: 337-9.
[84] Kiessling AA, Fitzgerald LM, Zhang D, *et al.* Human immunodeficiency virus in semen arises from a genetically distinct virus reservoir. *AIDS Res. Hum. Retroviruses* 1998; 14: 33-41.
[85] Barroso PF, Schechter M, Gupta P, *et al.* Effect of antiretroviral therapy on HIV shedding in semen. *Ann. Intern. Med.* 2000; 133: 280-4.
[86] Bujan L, Daudin M, Matsuda T, *et al.* Factors of intermittent HIV-1 excretion in semen and efficiency of sperm processing in obtaining spermatozoa without HIV-1 genomes. *AIDS* 2004; 18: 757-66.
[87] Leruez-Ville M, de Almeida M, Tachet A, *et al.* Assisted reproduction in HIV-1-serodifferent couples: the need for viral validation of processed semen. *AIDS* 2002; 16: 2267-73.
[88] Taylor S, Back DJ, Drake SM, *et al.* Antiretroviral drug concentrations in semen of HIV-infected men: differential penetration of indinavir, ritonavir and saquinavir. *J. Antimicrob. Chemother.* 2001; 48: 351-4.
[89] Davey RT, Jr, Bhat N, Yoder C, Chun TW, Metcalf JA, Dewar R, et al. Hiv-1 and t cell dynamics after interruption of highly active antiretroviral therapy (haart) in patients with a history of sustained viral suppression. *Proceedings of the National Academy of Sciences of the United States of America.* 1999;96:15109–15114
[90] Anderson DJ, O'Brien TR, Politch JA, *et al.* Effects of disease stage and zidovudine therapy on the detection of human immunodeficiency virus type 1 in semen. *JAMA* 1992; 267: 2769-74.
[91] Taylor B, Taylor S, Ferguson NM, Cane PA, *et al.* Dynamics of seminal plasma HIV-1 decline after antiretroviral treatment. *AIDS* 2001; 15: 424-6.
[92] Robbinson WA, Witt KL, Haseman JK, *et al.* Antiretroviral therapy effects on genetic and morphologic end points in lymphocytes and sperm of men with human immunodeficiency virus infection. *J. Infect. Dis.* 2001; 184: 127-35.
[93] Yeni PG, Hammer SM, Carpenter CC, *et al.* Antiretroviral treatment for adult HIV infection in 2002: updated recommendations of the International AIDS Society-USA Panel. *JAMA* 2002; 288: 222-35.
[94] White DJ, Mital D, Taylor S, St John JC. Sperm mitochondrial DNA deletions as a consequence of long term highly active antiretroviral therapy. AIDS 2001; 15: 1061-2.
[95] Diehl S, Vernazza P, Trein A, *et al.* Mitochondrial DNA and sperm quality in patients under antiretroviral therapy. *AIDS* 2003; 17: 450-1.
[96] Royce RA, Seña A, Cates W Jr, Cohen MS. Sexual transmission of HIV. *N. Engl. J. Med.* 1997; 336: 1072-8.
[97] Peterman TA, Stoneburner RL, Allen JR, Jaffe HW, Curran JW. Risk of human immunodeficiency virus transmission from heterosexual adults with transfusion-associated infections. *JAMA* 1988; 259: 55-8.
[98] de Vincenzi I. A longitudinal study of human immunodeficiency virus transmission by heterosexual partners. European Study Group on Heterosexual Transmission of HIV. *N. Engl. J. Med.* 1994; 331: 341-6.

[99] Gray RH, Wawer MJ, Brookmeyer R, *et al.* Probability of HIV-1 transmission per coital act in monogamous, heterosexual, HIV-1- discordant couples in Rakai, Uganda. *Lancet* 2001; 357: 1149-53.

[100] Cameron DW, Simonsen JN, D'Costa LJ, *et al.* Female to male transmission of human immunodeficiency virus type 1: risk factors for seroconversion in men. *Lancet* 1989; 2: 403-7.

[101] Mastro TD, Satten GA, Nopkesorn T, Sangkharomya S, Longini IM Jr. Probability of female-to-male transmission of HIV-1 in Thailand. *Lancet* 1994; 343: 204-7.

[102] Zunzunegui V, Casabona J, Laguna J, *et al.* Risk factors for the heterosexual transmission of HIV from man to woman: a Spanish multicenter study. *Med. Clin.* (Barc.) 1992; 98: 721-5.

[103] Attia S, Egger M, Müller M, Zwahlen M, Low N. Sexual transmission of HIV according to viral load and antiretroviral therapy: systematic review and meta-analysis. *AIDS 2009;* 23:1397–1404.

[104] Vernazza PL, Eron JJ, Fiscus SA, Cohen MS. Sexual transmisi6n of HIV: infectiousness and prevention. *AIDS* 1999; 13: 155-66.

[105] Granich RM, Gilks CF, Dye C, De Cock KM, Williams BG. Universal voluntary HIV testing with immediate antiretroviral therapy as a strategy for elimination of HIV transmission: a mathematical model. *Lance 2009;*, 373:48–57.

[106] Delvaux T, Nöstlinger C. Reproductive choice for women and men living with HIV: contraception, abortion and fertility. *Reprod. Health Matters* 2007; 15: 46-66.

[107] Public Health Service Task Force. Recommendations for use of Antiretroviral drugs in pregnant HIV-1 infected women for maternal health and interventions to reduce perinatal HIV-1 transmission in the United States. July 8 2008.

[108] de Ruiter A, Mercey D, Anderson J, *et al.* British HIV Association and Children's HIV Association guidelines for the management of HIV infection in pregnant women 2008. *HIV Med.* 2008; 9: 452- 502.

[109] Gilling -Smith C. HIV prevention. Assisted reproduction in HIVdiscordant couples. *AIDS Read* 2000; 10: 581-7.

[110] Rouzioux C, Costagliola D, Burgard M, *et al.* Estimated timing of mother-to-child human immunodeficiency virus type 1 (HIV-1) transmission by use of a Markov model. The HIV Infection in Newborns French Collaborative Study Group. *Am. J. Epidemiol.* 1995; 15: 142: 1330-7.

[111] Reproduction in couples with chronic viral infections. ce comm J, Vidal C, Fortuño S, Bellver J. *Current women's health reviews* 2009; 5: 130-48.

[112] van Leeuwen E, Prins JM, Jurriaans S, *et al.* Reproduction and fertility in human immunodeficiency virus type-1 infection. *Hum. Reprod. Update* 2007; 13: 197-206.

[113] Ohl J, Partisani M, Wittemer C, *et al.* Encouraging results despite complexity of multidisciplinary care of HIV-infected women using assisted reproduction techniques. *Hum. Reprod.* 2005; 20: 3136-40.

[114] The Practice Committee of the American Society for reproductive Medicine. Guidelines for reducing the risk of viral transmission during fertility treatment. *Fertil. Steril.* 2008; 90: 156-62.

[115] Manigart Y, Rozenberg S, Barlow P, *et al.* ART outcome in HIVinfected patients. *Hum. Reprod.* 2006; 11: 2935-40.

[116] Sturt AS, Dokubo EK, Sint TT. Antiretroviral therapy (ART) for treating HIV infection in ART-eligible pregnant women. *Cochrane Database Syst. Rev.* 2010 Mar 17;(3):CD008440.

[117] Newell ML, Pembrey L: Mother-to-child transmission of hepatitis C virus infection. *Hepatology* 2002: 36: 106-13.

[118] Gilling-Smith C, Almeida P; Practice and Policy Committee of the British Fertility Society. HIV, hepatitis B and hepatitis C and infertility: reducing risk. *Hum. Fertil. (Camb)* 2003; 6: 106-12.

[119] Quinn TC, Wawer MJ, Sewankambo N, *et al.* Viral load and heterosexual transmission of human immunodeficiency virus type 1. Rakai Project Study Group. N *Engl. J. Med.* 2000; 342: 921-9.

[120] Peña JE, Thornton MH, Sauer MV. Complications of *in vitro* fertilization with intracytoplasmic sperm injection in human immunodeficiency virus serodiscordant couples. *Arch. Gynecol. Obstet.* 2003; 268: 198-201.

[121] Guilbert J, Merlet F, LeDu A, *et al.* ICSI for HIV-1 serodifferent couples: results of a preliminary study. *Hum. Reprod.* 2001; 17: 56-7.

[122] Weigel MM, Kremer H, Sonnenberg-Schwan U, *et al.* Diagnostics and treatment of HIV-discordant couples who wish to have children. *Eur. J. Med. Res.* 2001; 6: 317-21.

[123] Scavalli CP, Mandelbrot L, Berrebi A, *et al.* Twin pregnancy as a risk factor for mother-to-child transmission of HIV-1: trends over 20 years. *AIDS 2007*; 21: 993-1002.

[124] Terriou P, Auquier P, Chabert-Orsini V, *et al.* Outcome of ICSI in HIV-1-infected women. *Hum. Reprod.* 2005; 20: 2838-43.

[125] Coll O, Suy A, Figueras F, *et al.* Decreased pregnancy rate after invitro fertilization in HIV-infected women receiving HAART. *AIDS 2006*; 20: 121-3.

[126] Martinet V, Manigart Y, Rozenberg S, Becker B, Gerard M, Delvigne A. Ovarian response to stimulation of HIV-positive

[127] López S, Coll O, Durban M, *et al.* Mitochondrial DNA depletion in oocytes of HIV-infected antiretroviral-treated infertile women. *Antivir. Ther.* 2008; 13: 833-8.

[128] Chan DJ, Ray JE, McNally L, Batterham M, Smith DE. Correlation between HIV-1 RNA load in blood and seminal plasma depending on antiretroviral treatment status, regimen and penetration of semen by antiretroviral drugs. *Current HIV Research.* 2008;6:477–484.

[129] Ghosn J, Chaix ML, Peytavin G, Bresson JL, Galimand J, Girard PM, Raffi F, Cohen-Codar I, Delfraissy JF, Rouzioux C. Absence of HIV-1 shedding in male genital tract after 1 year of first-line lopinavir/ritonavir alone or in combination with zidovudine/lamivudine. *Journal of Antimicrobial Chemotherapy.* 2008;61:1344–1347

[130] Vernazza P, Daneel S, Schiffer V, Decosterd L, Fierz W, Klimkait T, Hoffmann M, Hirschel B. The role of compartment penetration in PI-monotherapy: the Atazanavir-Ritonavir Monomaintenance (ATARITMO) Trial. *AIDS. 2007*;21:1309–1315.

[131] Marcelin AG, Tubiana R, Lambert-Niclot S, Lefebvre G, Dominguez S, Bonmarchand M, et al. Detection of HIV-1 RNA in seminal plasma samples from treated patients with undetectable HIV-1 RNA in blood plasma. *AIDS. 2008*;22:1677–1679

[132] Pasquier CJ, Moinard N, Saune K, Souyris C, Lavit M, Daudin M, Izopet J, Bujan L. Persistent differences in the antiviral effects of highly active antiretroviral therapy in the blood and male genital tract. *AIDS. 2008*;22:1894–1896

[133] Barreiro P, Castilla JA, Labarga P, Soriano V. Is natural conception a valid option for HIV-serodiscordant couples?. *Hum. Reprod. 2007*; 22: 2353-8.
[134] Barreiro P, del Romero J, Leal M, *et al.* Spanish HIV- Discordant Study Group. Natural pregnancies in HIV-serodiscordant couples receiving successful antiretroviral therapy. *J. Acquir. Immune Deficit. Syndr*. 2006; 43: 324-6.
[135] Vernazza P, Hirschel B, Bernasconi E, Flepp M. HIV seropositive persons without sexually transmitted diseases under fully suppressive antiretroviral treatment do not sexually transmit HIV. *Bulletin des médecins Suisses*. 2008;89:165–169.
[136] A Le Tortorec and N Dejucq-Rainsford. HIV infection of the male genital tract – consequences for sexual transmission and reproduction *Int. J. Androl.* 2010 February; 33(1): e98–e108.
[137] Vandermaelen A, Englert Y. Human immunodeficiency virus serodiscordant couples on highly active antiretroviral therapies with undetectable viral load: conception by unprotected sexual intercourse or by assisted reproduction techniques?.]. *Hum. Reprod.* 2010 Feb;25(2):374-9.
[138] Nicopoullos JD, Almeida P, Vourliotis M, Goulding R, Gilling-Smith C. A decade of sperm washing: clinical correlates of successful insemination outcome. *Hum. Reprod.* 2010 Aug;25(8):1869-76.
[139] Nicopoullos JD, Almeida P, Vourliotis M, Gilling-Smith C. A decade of the sperm-washing programme: correlation between markers of HIV and seminal parameters. *HIV Med*. 2010 Aug 17. [Epub ahead of print].
[140] Marina S, Marina F, Alcolea R, *et al.* Pregnancy following intracytoplasmic sperm injection from an HIV-1-seropositive man. Hum Reprod 1998; 13: 3247-9.
[141] Meseguer M, Garrido N, Gimeno C, *et al.* Comparison of polymerase chain reaction-dependent methods for determining the presence of human immunodeficiency virus and hepatitis C virus in washed sperm. Comparison of polymerase chain reactiondependent methods for determining the presence of human immunodeficiency virus and hepatitis C virus in washed sperm. *Fertil. Steril.* 2002; 78: 1199-202.
[142] Garrido N, Meseguer M, Bellver J, Remohi J, Simon C, Pellicer A. Report of the results of a 2 year programme of sperm wash and ICSI treatment for human immunodeficiency virus and hepatitis C virus serodiscordant couples. *Hum. Reprod.* 2004; 19: 2581-6.
[143] Semprini AE, Levi-Setti P, Bozzo M, *et al.* Insemination of HIVnegative women with processed semen of HIV-positive partners. *Lancet* 1992; 340: 1317-9.
[144] Semprini AE, Fiore S, Pardi G. Reproductive counselling for HIVdiscordant couples. *Lancet* 1997; 349: 1401-2.
[145] Marina S, Marina F, Alcolea R, *et al.* Human immunodeficiency virus type 1--serodiscordant couples can bear healthy children after undergoing intrauterine insemination. *Fertil. Steril.* 1998; 70: 35-9.
[146] Tur R, Veiga A, Busquets A, *et al.* Artificial insemination with processed sperm samples from serodiscordant couples for HIV-1. *Hum. Reprod*. 1999; 14: 208.
[147] Semprini AE: Viral transmission in ART: risk for patients and health care providers. *Hum. Reprod*. 2000; 15: abstract 69.
[148] Gilmour JW, Gilling-Smith C, Gotch F. Reduction of HIV transmission in HIV-discordant couples wishing to conceive. *AIDS 2001*; 15: 429-30.
[149] Bujan L, Daudin M, Pasquier C. Reproductive options for HIVserodiscordant couples. *Perspect Sex Reprod Health 2002*; 34: 104.

[150] Quintana R, Tiveron M, Garcia F, Kopcow L, Bisioli C, Young E. Intrauterine insemination (IUI), *in vitro* fertilization (IVF) and intracytoplasmic sperm injection (ICSI) in human immunodeficiency virus (HIV) serodiscordant couples: results and perpectives. *Fertil. Steril.* 2002; 78: 116.
[151] Ohl J, Partisani M, Wittemer C, *et al.* Assisted reproduction techniques for HIV serodiscordant couples: 18 months of experience. *Hum. Reprod.* 2003; 18: 1244-9.
[152] Bujan L, Pasquier C, Labeyrie E, Lanusse-Crousse P, Morucci M, Daudin M. Insemination with isolated and virologically tested spermatozoa is a safe way for human immunodeficiency type 1 virus-serodiscordant couples with an infected male partner to have a child. *Fertil. Steril.* 2004; 82: 857-62.
[153] Peña JE, Thornton MH, Sauer MV. Assessing the clinical utility of *in vitro* fertilization with intracytoplasmic sperm injection in human immunodeficiency virus type 1 serodiscordant couples: report of 113 consecutive cycles. *Fertil. Steril.* 2003; 80: 356-62.
[154] Savasi V, Ferrazzi E, Lanzani C, Oneta M, Parrilla B, Persico T. Safety of sperm washing and ART outcome in 741 HIV-1- serodiscordant couples. *Hum. Reprod.* 2007; 22: 772-7.
[155] Melo MA, Meseguer M, Bellver J, *et al.* Human immunodeficiency type-1 virus (HIV-1) infection in serodiscordant couples (SDCs) does not have an impact on embryo quality or intracytoplasmic sperm injection (ICSI) outcome. *Fertil. Steril.* 2008; 89: 141-50.
[156] Garrido N, Gil-Salom M, Martínez-Jabaloyas JM, Meseguer M. First report of the absence of viral load in testicular sperm samples obtained from men with hepatitis C and HIV after washing and their subsequent use. *Fertil. Steril.* 2009 Sep;92(3):1012-5.
[157] Savasi V, Ferrazzi E, Lanzani C, Oneta M, Parrilla B, Persico T. Safety of sperm washing and ART outcome in 741 HIV-1- serodiscordant couples. *Hum. Reprod.* 2007; 22: 772-7.
[158] Sauer MV, Choi J. HIV seroconversion in a woman preparing for assisted reproduction: an inherent risk in caring for HIVserodiscordant copules. *Reprod. Biomed. Online* 2006; 12: 375-7.
[159] Chu MC, Peña JE, Nakhuda GS, Thornton MH 2nd, Sauer MV. Assessing the reproductive performance of men co-infected with HIV-1 and hepatitis C undergoing assisted reproduction. *Arch. Gynecol. Obstet.* 2006; 274: 155-9.
[160] Shepard CW, Simard EP, Finelli L, Fiore AE, Bell BP. Hepatitis B virus infection: epidemiology and vaccination. *Epidemiol. Rev.* 2006; 28: 112-25.
[161] The Practice Committee of the American Society for Reproductive Medicine. Hepatitis and reproduction. *Fertil. and Steril.* 2008; 90: 226-35.
[162] Smith D. Preconception counselling for patients with chronical viral hepatitis. *Postgrad. Obstet. Gynecol.* 2005; 25: 1-10.
[163] Van Herck K, Van Damme P. Benefits of early hepatitis B immunization programs for newborns and infants. *Pediatr. Infect. Dis. J.* 2008; 27: 861-9.
[164] Bacq Y. Hepatitis B and pregnancy. *Gastroenterol. Clin. Biol.* 2008; 32: 12-9.
[165] Baker DA, Mead PB, Hager WD. Hepatitis B infection in pregnancy. Protocols for infectious diseases in obstetrics and gynecology. *Blackwell Sci.* 2000: 204-14.
[166] Michielsen PP, van Damme P. Viral hepatitis and pregnancy. *Acta Gastroenterol. Belg.* 1999; 62: 21-9.

[167] Pawlotsky JM. Assisted reproduction and viral hepatitis: the virologist's viewpoint. *Contracept. Fertil. Sex* 1997; 25: 530-3.

[168] Wang S, Peng G, Li M, Xiao H, Jiang P, Zeng N, et al. Identification of hepatitis B virus vertical transmission from father to fetus by direct sequencing. Southeast Asian *J. Trop. Med. Public Health* 2003;34: 106–13.

[169] Lam PM, Suen SH, Lao TT, Cheung LP, Leung TY, et al. Hepatitis B infection and outcomes of in vitro fertilization and embryo transfer treatment. *Fertil. Steril.* 2010 Feb;93(2):480-5.

[170] American Academy of Pediatrics and the American college of Obstetricians and Gynecologist. Perinatal infections. Guidelines for perinatal care. 5th ed. 2002; 287-92.

[171] Hsu HM, Chen DS, Chuang CH. Efficacy of a mass hepatitis B vaccination program in Taiwan: studies on 3464 infants of hepatitis B surface antigen-carrier mothers. *JAMA* 1988; 224: 359-62.

[172] Wang Z, Zhang J, Yang H, *et al.* Quantitative analysis of HBV DNA level and HBeAg titer in hepatitis B surface antigen positive mothers and their babies: HBeAg passage through the placenta and the rate of decay in babies. *J. Med. Virol.* 2003; 71: 360-6.

[173] Lee SD, Lo KJ, Tsai YT, Wu JC. Maternal hepatitis B virus DNA in mother-infant transmission. *Lancet* 1989; 1: 719.

[174] Centers for Disease Control. Hepatitis B Virus: a comprehensive strategy for eliminінating transmission in the United States through universal childhood vaccination:recommendation s of the inmunization practices advisory committee (ACIP). *Morbid. Mortal. Wkly. Rep.* 1991; 40: 1-19.

[175] Gupta I, Ratho RK. Immunogenicity and safety of two schedules of Hepatitis B vaccination during pregnancy. *J. Obstet. Gynaecol. Res.* 2003; 29: 84-6.

[176] Sur DK, Wallis DH, O'Connell TX. Vaccinations in pregnancy. *Am. Fam. Physician.* 2003; 68: 299-304.

[177] Ye F, Yue Y, Li S, Chen T, Bai G, Liu M, et al. Presence of HBsAg, HBcAg, and HBV DNA in ovary and ovum of the patients with chronic hepatitis B virus infection. *Am. J. Obstet. Gynecol.* 2006;194:387–92.

[178] Kalu E, Wood R, Vourliotis M, Gilling-Smith C. Fertility needs and funding in couples with blood-borne viral infection. *HIV Med.* 2010 Jan;11(1):90-3.

[179] Lang ZW Distribution of hepatitis B virus in testicle tissue in patients with hepatitis B infection. . *Zhonghua Yi Xue Za Zhi* 1993; 73: 329-31, 379.

[180] Hadchouel M, Scotto J, Huret JL, *et al.* Presence of HBV DNA in spermatozoa: a possible vertical transmission of HBV *via* the germ line. *J. Med. Virol.* 1985; 16: 61-6.

[181] Lorusso F, Palmisano M, Chironna M, Vacca M, Masciandaro P, et al. Impact of chronic viral diseases on semen parameters. *Andrologia.* 2010 Apr;42(2):121-6.

[182] Lee VC, Ng EH, Yeung WS, Ho PC. Impact of positive hepatitis B surface antigen on the outcome of IVF treatment. *Reprod. Biomed. Online.* 2010 Nov;21(5):712-7.

[183] Pirwany I, Phillips S, Kelly S, Buckett W, Tan S. Reproductive performance of couples discordant for hepatitis B and C following IVF treatment. *J. Assist. Reprod. Genet.* 2004 May;21(5):157-61.

[184] McHutchison JG, Gordon SC, Schiff ER. Interferon alpha-2b alone or in combination with ribavirin as inicial treatment for chronic hepatitis c: Hepatitis Interventional Therapy Group. *N. Engl. J. Med.* 1998; 339: 1485-92.

[185] Airoldi J, Berghella V. Hepatitis C and pregnancy. *Obstet. Gynecol. Surv*. 2006; 61: 666-72.

[186] Paternoster DM, Santarossa C, Grella P, *et al*. Viral load in HCV RNA-positive pregnant women. *Am. J. Gastroenterol*. 2001; 96: 2751-4.

[187] Alter MJ. Epidemiology of hepatitis C in West. Semin Liver Dis 1995; 15: 5-14.

[188] Zuccotti GV, Ribero ML, Giovannini M, *et al*. Effect of hepatitis C genotype on mother-to-infant transmission of virus. *J. Pediatr*. 1995; 127: 278-80.

[189] Mok J, Pembrey L, Tovo PA, Newell ML. When does mother to child transmission of hepatitis C virus occur?. *Arch. Dis. Child Fetal Neonatal. Ed*. 2005; 90: 156-60.

[190] Resti M, Azzari C, Galli L, Zuin G, *et al*. Maternal drug use is a preeminent risk factor for mother-to-child hepatitis C virus transmission: results from a multicenter study of 1372 motherinfant pairs. *J. Infect. Dis*. 2002; 185: 567-72.

[191] Pergam SA, Wang CC, Gardella CM. Pregnancy complications associated with hepatitis C: data from a 2003-2005 Washington state birth cohort. *Am. J. Obstet. Gynecol*. 2008; 199: 38.e1-9.

[192] Levy R, Tardy JC, Bourlet T, *et al*. Transmission risk of hepatitis C virus in assisted reproductive techniques. *Hum. Reprod*. 2000; 15: 810-6.

[193] Keck C, Gerber-Schafer C, Clad A, *et al*. Seminal tract infections: impact on male fertility and treatment options. *Hum. Reprod. Update* 1998; 4: 891-903.

[194] Tohme RA, Holmberg SD. Is sexual contact a major mode of hepatitis C virus transmission? *Hepatology*. 2010 Oct;52(4):1497-505.

[195] Wang CC, Cook L, Tapia KA, Holte S, Krows M, Bagabag A, Santos A, Corey L, Jerome KR. Cervicovaginal shedding of hepatitis C viral RNA is associated with the presence of menstrual or other blood in cervicovaginal fluids. *J. Clin. Virol*. 2010 Oct 14. [Epub ahead of print].

[196] Dienstag JL. Sexual and perinatal transmission of hepatitis C. *Hepatology* 1997; 26: 66-70.

[197] Englert Y, Moens E. Imparired ovarian stimulation during *in vitro* fertilization in women who are seropositive for hepatitis C virus and seronegative for human immunodeficiency virus. *Fertil. Steril*. 2007; 88: 607-11.

[198] McKee TA, Avery S, Majid A, Brinsden PR. Risks for transmission of hepatitis C virus during artificial insemination. *Fertil. Steril*. 1996; 66: 161-3.

[199] Prisant N, Tubiana R, Lefebvre G, Lebray P, Marcelin AG, et al. HIV-1 or hepatitis C chronic infection in serodiscordant infertile couples has no impact on infertility treatment outcome. *Fertil. Steril*. 2010 Feb;93(3):1020-3.

[200] Foster Gr. Past, present and future hepatitis C treatments. *Semen. Liver Dis*. 2004; 24: 97-104.

[201] Cassuto NG, Sifer C, Feldmann G, *et al*. A modified RT-PCR technique to screen for viral RNA in the semen of hepatitis C viruspositive men. *Hum. Reprod*. 2002; 17: 3153-6.

[202] Honeck P, Weigel M, Kwon ST, Alken P, Bross S. Assisted procreation in cases of hepatitis B, hepatitis C or human immunodeficiency virus infection of the male partner. *Hum. Reprod*. 2006; 21: 1117-21.

[203] Narayana K, D'Souza UJ, Seetharama Rao KP. Ribavirin-induced sperm shape abnormalities in Wistar rat. *Mutat. Res*. 2002; 513:193- 6.

[204] Devaux A, Soula V, Sifer C, *et al.* Hepatitis C virus detection in follicular fluid and culture media from HCV+ women, and viral risk during IVF procedures. *Hum. Reprod.* 2003; 18: 2342-9.

[205] Taylor PJ, Gill MJ, Mahadevan M, Pattinson HA. Hepatitis B virus in human follicular fluid. *Fertil. Steril.* 1987; 48: 514.

[206] Gilling-Smith C, Emiliani S, Almeida P, Liesnard C, Englert Y. Laboratory safety during assisted reproduction in patients with blood-borne viruses. *Hum. Reprod.* 2005; 20: 1433-8.

[207] Bielanski A, Vajta G. Risk of contamination of germplasm during cryopreservation and cryobanking in IVF units. *Hum. Reprod.* 2009 Oct;24(10):2457-67.

[208] Pomeroy KO, Harris S, Conaghan J, Papadakis M, Centola G, et al. Storage of cryopreserved reproductive tissues: evidence that cross-contamination of infectious agents is a negligible risk. *Fertil. Steril.* 2010 Sep;94(4):1181-8.

[209] Tedder RS, Zuckerman MA, Goldstone AH, Hawkins AE, Fielding A, et al. Hepatitis B transmission from contaminated cryopreservation tank. *Lance*t 1995;346:137–40.

[210] Letur-K€onirsch H, Collin G, Sifer C, Devaux A, Kuttenn F, Madelenat P, et al. Safety of cryopreservation straws for human gametes or embryos: a study with human immunodeficiency virus-1 under cryopreservation conditions. *Hum. Reprod.* 2003;18:140–4.

[211] Implementing Directive 2004/23 EC of the European Parliamentand of the Council as regards traceably requirements, notificacion of serious adverse reaction and events and certain technical requirements for the coding, processing, preservation, storage and distribution of human tissues and cells. Comission Directive 2006/86 EC. *Official Journal of the European Union* 24 October 2006.

[212] Letur-Könirsch H, Collin G, Sifer C, *et al.* Safety of cryopreservation straws for human gametes or embryos: a study with human immunodeficiency virus-1 under cryopreservation conditions. *Hum. Reprod.* 2003; 18: 140-4.

[213] Balaban B, Yakin K, Isiklar A, Urman B. Utilization of high-security straws for embryo freezing in an in vitro fertilization program: a prospective, randomized study. *Fertil. Steril.* 2007 Mar;87(3):691-6.

[214] Bielanski A. Non-transmission of bacterial and viral microbes to embryos and semen stored in the vapour phase of liquid nitrogen in dry shippers. *Cryobiology.* 2005 Apr;50(2):206-10.

In: In Vitro Fertilization
Editor: Samantha P. Steiger, pp. 35-63
ISBN 978-1-61209-961-3

Chapter II

Intracytoplasmic Sperm Injection in Cattle

***Shinichi Hochi*[1], *Hany Abdalla*[1,2] and *Masumi Hirabayashi*[3]**
[1]Faculty of Textile Science and Technology, Shinshu University, Ueda, Nagano, Japan
[2]Faculty of Veterinary Medicine, Zagazig University, Zagazig, Sharkia, Egypt
[3]National Institute for Physiological Sciences, Okazaki, Aichi, Japan

Abstract

This chapter deals with intracytoplasmic sperm injection (ICSI) in domestic cattle. Following a brief review on the history of bovine ICSI and the technical aspects of piezo-ICSI, abilities of bovine embryos derived from ICSI and in vitro fertilization (IVF) are comparatively described as recent progress, with special references to active DNA demethylation of pronuclear zygotes, yield and quality of blastocysts, and their cryotolerance. Paternal genome is subjected to replication-independent, genome-wide active demethylation during the early phase after fertilization. Immunofluorescent analysis using anti-5-methylcytosine indicated that paternal genome rapidly demethylated within 10 hours after IVF and 6 hours after ICSI. The demethylation extent in pronuclear zygotes was moderate with $0.4 \leq RM < 0.6$ (RM: relative methylation, paternal methylation level relative to maternal counterpart). Due to the inability of the mechanical stimulation and/or the injected spermatozoon itself to induce proper oocyte activation after ICSI, exogenous activation treatments, such as ionomycin, ethanol, ionomycin + cycloheximide, or ionomycin + 6-dimethylaminopurine, have been applied to ICSI oocytes. Based on a direct comparative study, a new activation regimen composed from two triggers for single calcium increase (5 μM ionomycin for 5 min immediately after ICSI plus 7% ethanol for 5 min 4 hours after ICSI) without using either protein synthesis or protein phosphorylation inhibitors was proposed. While 40% of IVF oocytes reached blastocysts until Day-8, approximately 30% of ICSI oocytes activated with ionomycin + ethanol were able to develop into blastocysts. Such blastocysts were subjected to minimum volume cooling vitrification procedure using Cryotop as cryodevice. Post-warming survival of ICSI-derived fully-expanded blastocysts was similar to that of their IVF-derived counterparts. However, the ability of ICSI-derived expanding blastocysts to survive the vitrification procedures was lower than that of IVF-derived blastocysts, although the ICSI- and IVF-derived fresh blastocysts were of similar quality.

Introduction

Many advanced / assisted reproductive technologies (ART) are applied in the field of animal reproduction for different purposes. Those originally developed in the decades from 1950's to 1970's include artificial insemination and multiple ovulations and embryo transfer with or without cryopreservation of spermatozoa and preimplantation-stage embryos. Since the latest few decades (1980's-), in vitro production of transferable embryos by in vitro fertilization (IVF) has become practical not only in small experimental animals but also the large domestic species. Some more complicated techniques have been applied to facilitate the access of sperm cells to oolemma through the zona pellucida (ZD: zona-drilling, ZO: zona-opening, PZD: partial zona dissection), to escape the capacitation- / acrosome reaction-based penetration of sperm cells into the zona (SUZI: subzonal sperm injection), or to escape the spontaneous penetration of paternal gametes into the ooplasm (ICSI: intracytoplasmic sperm injection, ELSI: elongating spermatid injection, ROSI: round spermatid injection). Even production of viable offspring without using sperm cells as paternal gametes (SCNT: somatic cell nuclear transfer) was proven in many mammalian species during this decade, while nuclear transfer of embryonic blastomeres has already resulted in the successful birth of cloned sheep and cattle in the late 1970's.

After fertilization, each gamete (spermatozoa / oocyte) participates into some well-organized post-fertilization events essential for physiological embryonic development, including sperm-induced oocyte activation, remodeling of paternal genome, microtubule organization for fusion of both pronuclei, epigenetic remodeling, and activation of embryonic genome. Some of these events may be disturbed after application of some ART, and subsequent embryonic development to the blastocyst stage may be affected.

1. Background

1.1. Application and History of Bovine ICSI

Direct injection of a spermatozoon into ooplasm (homogenous ICSI) is used not only to investigate the fundamental aspects around fertilization, but also to overcome some forms of male infertility in human (Vernaeve et al., 2003). The ICSI technique is applicable for offspring production from immotile spermatozoa (freeze-dried sperm, sperm frozen without cryoprotection, or testicular sperm), and also for production of transgenic animals using exogenous DNA-bound spermatozoa (Perry et al., 1999a; Hirabayashi et al., 2005a). Interspecies ICSI using oocytes from laboratory or domestic species is effective to analyze some functions of human spermatozoa (Rybouchkin et al., 1995; Nakamura et al., 2001). Further advantages of ICSI are its ability to overcome the low fertilization rate or polyspermic penetration in cryopreserved oocytes (Vincent et al., 1990; Rho et al., 2004) and the limited number and lowered motility in the flow-cytometrically sorted, sex-determined spermatozoa (Hamano et al., 1999). In bovine, the ICSI technique can be applied to achieve the best utilization of genetically superior males characterized by low sperm cell concentration, low motility in their ejaculate or poor or suboptimal reaction with the in vitro capacitation process required for IVF protocol (Ushijima and Nakane, 2006).

Table 1. Summary for bovine ICSI studies conducted during the latest decade

ICSI protocol	Oocyte activation	Sperm treatment	% Cleavage	% Blastocysts	% Offspring	References
	Non	DTT	3	0	---	
Conv.	Io	DTT	17	4	---	Rho et al. (1998a)
	Io+6-DMAP*	DTT	61	24	---	
Conv.	EtOH (x1-2)	Sonicated, sorted head	14–48	4–7	21 (10/48)	Hamano et al. (1999)
Conv	Ca-ionophore	FT	52	13	---	Keskintepe and Brackett (2000)
Piezo	Non	FT	40–74	3–5	---	Emuta and Horiuchi (2001)
	EtOH	FT	65–70	7–21	---	
	Non	Repeated FT	15	0	---	
Piezo	EtOH	Repeated FT	28	1	---	Horiuchi et al. (2002)
	Non	Tail scoring	63	8	---	
	EtOH	Tail scoring	70	15	50 (5/10)	
Piezo	Non	Tail cutting	72	23	57 (4/7) Day-60 pregnancy	Wei and Fukui (2002)
	Non	DTT	3	0	---	
Conv.	Io	DTT	17	1	---	Ock et al. (2003)
	Io+6-DMAP	DTT	70	18	---	
	Io+6-DMAP*	DTT	67	15	---	
	Non	FT	59	15	---	
Piezo	Io	FT	51	6	---	Galli et al. (2003)
	Io+CHX	FT	60–67	17–21	17 (1/6)	
	Io+CHX	DTT	66	24	---	
Piezo	Non	FT	13	4	---	Fujinami et al. (2004)
	EtOH	FT	51	14	---	
Conv.	Io+CHX	DTT	70	16	---	Rho et al. (2004)
	Non	FT	48	8	---	
Piezo	Io	FT	58	18	---	Oikawa et al. (2005)
	Io+6-DMAP*	FT	84	40	9 (1/11)	
	EtOH	FT	76	29	47 (7/17)	
Piezo	Io+Roscovitine	FT	72	15	---	Devito et al. (2010)
Conv.	Io+Roscovitine	FT	67	0	---	

Offspring rate was calculated from transferred embryos as shown in parentheses.

Abbreviations; Conv.: Conventional, Io: Ionomycin, 6-DMAP: 6-dimethylaminopurine, EtOH: Ethanol, CHX: Cyclohexiamide, DTT: Dithiothreitol, FT: Freeze-thawed.

*Three-hours culture was inserted between the two chemical treatments in the activation regimen.

The first attempt of mammalian ICSI was reported in hamster by Uehara and Yanagimachi (1976). Since then, a lot of ICSI experiments have been conducted in different mammalian species, with the first successful birth of offspring derived from ICSI oocytes in rabbit (Hosoi et al., 1988), followed by cattle (Goto et al., 1990), human (Palermo et al., 1992), mouse (Kimura and Yanagimachi, 1995), sheep (Catt et al., 1996), cat (Pope et al., 1998), horse (Cochran et al., 1998), pig (Martin, 2000), rat (Hirabayashi et al., 2002) and hamster (Yamauchi et al., 2002). The success rate, assessed by in vitro and in vivo development after ICSI, is highly variable among mammalian species, with the highest success rate in human and mouse (Kimura and Yanagimachi, 1995; Neri et al., 2008). Since the first attempt of bovine ICSI (Westhusin et al., 1984), the developmental potential of the ICSI oocytes into blastocysts in vitro or live calves in vivo is still low, unstable and far from satisfactory regardless of the numerous efforts. A complete summary for bovine ICSI studies during the latest decade is shown in Table 1. So far, piezo-assisted sperm injection followed by ethanol treatment is likely to achieve the best blastocyst yield in vitro and full-term development after transfer into recipient cattle.

1.2. Technique of Bovine ICSI

Detailed procedure for bovine piezo-ICSI employed in our laboratory (Abdalla et al., 2009a) is shown in Figure 1. For preparation of the injection pipette, borosilicate glass capillaries (outer diameter=1 mm and inner diameter=0.75 mm; Sutter Instrument) were pulled on a mechanical micropipette puller (Sutter Instrument, P97/IVF) at the following setting of parameters; heat=775, pull=30, velocity=200 and time=80. The pulled capillary pipette was cut, at a point of 7-9 μm in the outer diameter, with microforge (Narishige Scientific Instrument, MF-900). The tip of the injection pipette was rinsed with 25% hydrofluoric acid for 5 sec and washed with Milli-Q water followed by 100% ethanol. The hydrofluoric acid digests the glass in the tip of the pipette to increase the inner diameter, without changing the outer diameter and increasing the sharpness of the pipette tip. A small volume of mercury (2-3 mm length in the pipette) was introduced into the wide opposite end of the injection pipette, and was pushed forward to the tapered end of the pipette. To prepare the holding pipette, a glass capillary with 1 mm in the outer diameter (Narishige Scientific Instrument) was pulled with a micropipette puller (Narishige Scientific instrument). The pulled capillary pipette was cut with an ampoule cutter, and then the tip of the pipette was fire-polished with a heated glass ball in the microforge. The holding pipette has an outer diameter of about 50 μm and an inner diameter of about 20 μm, with a bent angle of about 30° at the anterior part of the pipette.

Motile spermatozoa were separated by the percoll-washing and washed twice with BSA-free mBO solution for 5 min each at 300 × *g*. Immediately before the ICSI, 2 μL of the sperm suspension were mixed with 8 μL of M2 medium containing 10% PVP-360. The PVP solution was effective not only to slow down the motility of the sperm (thus facilitating the catching of the sperm) but also to act as a lubricant to avoid adhesion of the sperm into the inner surface of the injection pipette (thus facilitating the controlling the sperm by the injection pipette). The ICSI was performed with a piezo-driven micromanipulator (PMAS-CT150; PrimeTech, Ibaraki, Japan). Briefly, single spermatozoon was immobilized by applying several piezo pulses to the midpiece before being aspirated tail first into a blunt-ended injection pipette. An oocyte was held with the holding pipette as the polar body was located either at 6 or 12 o'clock position. The zona pellucida was drilled by several piezo pulses (speed 2, intensity 2). The spermatozoon was repositioned to the tip of the injection pipette, and the injection pipette was advanced mechanically deep into the center of the oocyte, stretching the oolemma extensively. Upon application of a single piezo pulse (speed 2, intensity 2), the oolemma was punctured at the pipette tip. The sperm was gently injected into the ooplasm and the injection pipette was withdrawn.

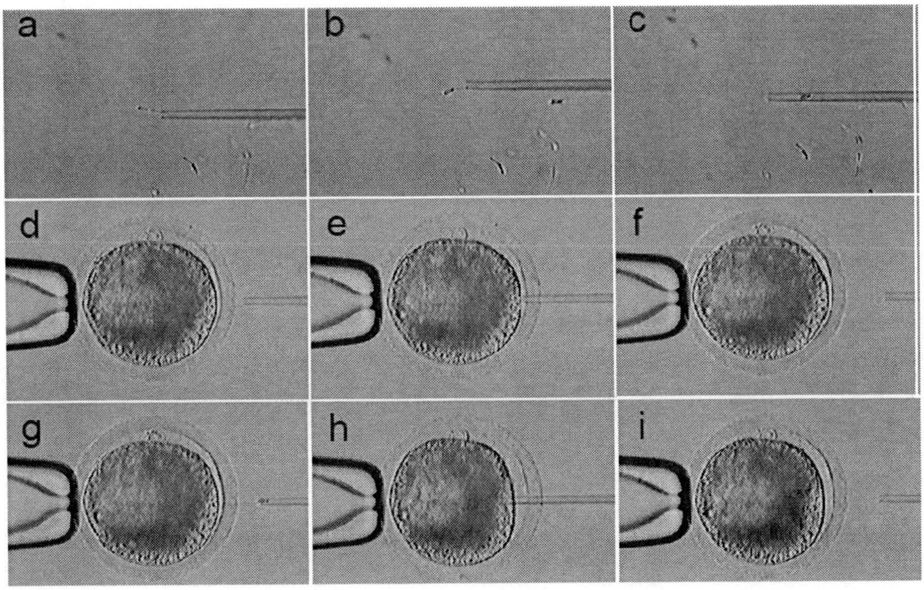

Figure 1. Intracytoplasmic sperm injection procedure in the bovine. (a) Catching a single spermatozoon: Make a sharp focus on the end piece of a motile spermatozoon, and control the injection pipette in X,Y and Z axis to be just behind the end piece. Then, aspirate the sperm tail first into the injection pipette. Motile spermatozoa are usually present in the bottom of the sperm droplet. (b) Immobilization of the spermatozoon: Adjust the sperm with the head outside and the midpiece touching to the tip of the injection pipette. Then, apply several piezo pulses until the sperm tail movement stops. (c) Re-positioning of the sperm: Aspirate the immobilized sperm into the injection pipette and bring it to the injection droplet containing the oocytes by moving the microscope stage. (d) Holding an oocyte to be injected: Make a sharp focus on an oocyte and Z-axis control of the holding pipette to approach the oocyte. Then, apply gentle suction into the holding pipette to catch the oocyte. Attention-1: The equatorial plane of the oocyte and the internal opening of the holding pipette must be in a same horizontal line. Attention-2: The polar body must be located either at 6 or 12 o'clock with positioning the largest perivitelline space at 3 o'clock area. Move the holding pipette to make both oocyte and spermatozoon present in a focus on X-axis. (e) Penetration of the zona pellucida: Access the injection pipette to touch the zona pellucida and apply a few piezo pulses. Attention-3: Avoid touching the relaxed plasma membrane by the injection pipette, if the pipette passed through the zona pellucida suddenly. (f) Removing of the zona core and re-positioning of the sperm: Move the injection pipette backward from the zona pellucida and release the zona core into the droplet. Then, re-position the sperm into near the tip of the injection pipette. If the zona was penetrated without aspirating the core into the injection pipette, the remaining core may disturb the subsequent operation for sperm microinjection. (g) Passing through zona pellucida: By the X-axis control, move the injection pipette with re-positioned sperm through the hole that has been made in the zona pellucida. (h) Penetration of the plasma membrane and injection of the sperm: Push forward the injection pipette against the plasma membrane until its tip is appeared to reach center of the oocytes. Then, apply a single piezo-pulse and push the pipette slightly forward while injecting the sperm. (i) Withdrawal of the injection pipette: Gently pull the injection pipette out of the oocyte.

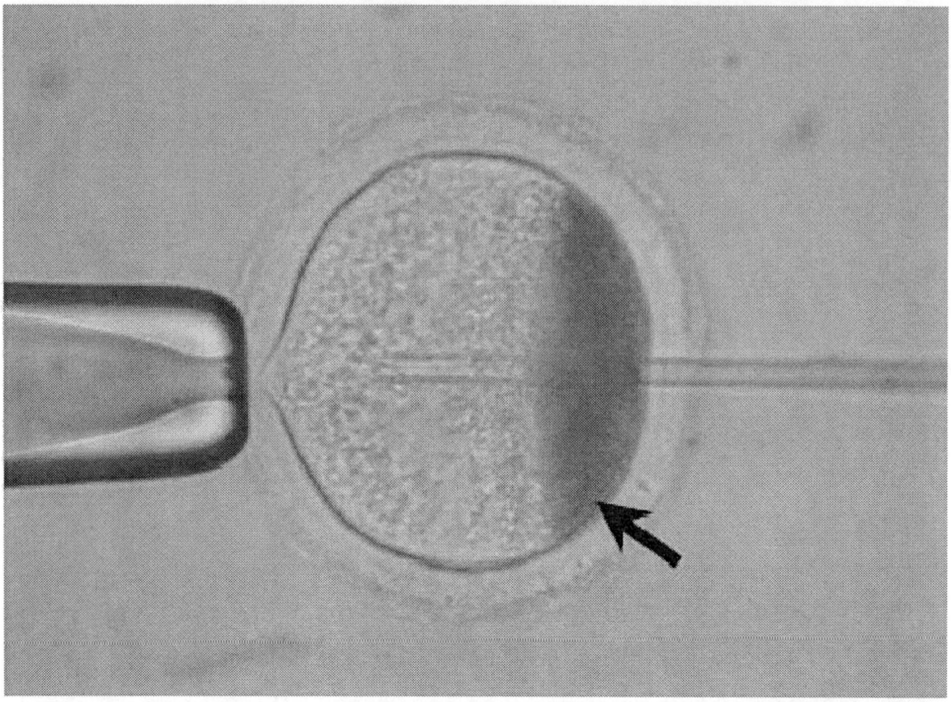

Figure 2. Sperm injection into a centrifuged bovine oocyte. High magnitude centrifugation of bovine oocytes makes it possible to localize the cytoplasmic lipids (arrow). By adjusting the area containing the localized lipids in the side facing to the injection pipette, the operator can visualize the tip of the injection pipette inside the clarified area of the cytoplasm. Thus, the rupture of the oolemma and the injection of sperm with minimum volume of the holding medium become easily recognizable.

Bovine oocytes appear dark because the ooplasm contains lipid droplets at a very high concentration. Centrifugation of bovine oocytes (600 x *g* for 7 min at an ambient temperature) makes it possible to localize the cytoplasmic lipids (Figure 2). By adjusting the area containing the localized lipids in the side facing to the injection pipette, the operator can visualize the tip of the injection pipette inside the clarified area of the cytoplasm. Therefore, the rupture of the oolemma and the injection of sperm with minimum volume of the holding medium become easily recognizable. Centrifugation of bovine oocytes *per se* does not have any adverse effects on the developmental potential of IVF-derived zygotes (Wall and Howk, 1988). Wei and Fukui (2000) reported that proportions of bovine oocytes successfully injected, survived or showed two pronuclei were higher when the centrifuged oocytes were used in conventional ICSI. However in our laboratory, application of oocyte centrifugation before piezo-ICSI did not improve the proportions of oocytes surviving the ICSI procedure (78 versus 83% in non-centrifuged group), extruding the polar body (52 versus 52%), cleaving (55 versus 50%), nor developing into blastocysts (15 versus 16%), under an activation treatment of ICSI oocytes with 7% ethanol for 5 min.

1.3. Possible Causes for Low Success in Bovine ICSI

Transferable bovine blastocysts can be produced in vitro either by co-culturing presumptive zygotes for >7 days with somatic cells such as oviductal epithelial cells or cumulus cells (Lu et al., 1988), or by culturing the zygotes under a lowered oxygen concentration (Bavister, 1995). During the culture period, the bovine zygotes undergo a risk of developmental block at the 8- to 16-cell stage where the pattern of genome activation changes from maternal to embryonic (maternal + paternal) sources (Telford et al., 1990; Barnes and First, 1991). The blastocyst yield from IVF-derived bovine zygotes is approximately 30–40%, while that from ICSI-derived zygotes is variable (5-40%). Characteristic phenomenon after bovine ICSI as (1) failure of oocytes activation, (2) compromised sperm chromatin remodeling, and (3) technical difficulties may be a possible reason for such a low success rate.

1.3.1. Failure of Oocyte Activation

Unlike the IVF-derived bovine oocytes, majority of bovine ICSI oocytes did not show any calcium oscillations, with a few oocytes showing a single transient increase (Malcuit et al., 2006b). Such abnormal response causes temporal inactivation followed by rapid re-accumulation of maturation-promoting factor (MPF) in ICSI oocytes (Fujinami et al., 2004). This accompanied with high proportion of ICSI oocytes either still arrested at the second meiotic division (M-II) or released from the M-II but re-arrested again at the so-called M-III before completing the second meiotic division (Chung et al., 2000). To overcome this problem, bovine ICSI oocytes were treated with mechanical or chemical stimuli to induce intracellular calcium spike such as direct current (Hwang et al., 2000), calcium ionophore (Keskintepe and Brackett, 2000), ionomycin (Rho et al., 1998a; Chung et al., 2000; Ock et al., 2003; Galli et al., 2003; Oikawa et al., 2005) or ethanol (Emuta and Horiuchi, 2002; Horiuchi et al., 2002; Oikawa et al., 2005). Since these stimuli did not induce a long-lasting oscillations (Hoth and Penner, 1992; Shiina et al., 1993), they have been combined with other chemicals that either interfere with the re-synthesis (a protein phosphorylation inhibitors; Cycloheximide, CHX; Galli et al., 2003; Rho et al., 2004) or the activation of the MPF (a protein phosphorylation inhibitors; 6-dimethylaminopurine, 6-DMAP; Rho et al., 1998a; Ock et al., 2003; Oikawa et al., 2005; a cyclin-dependent kinase inhibitor; Roscovitine; Devito et al., 2010). However, 6-DMAP interfered with chromosomal segregation and polar body extrusion which resulted in abnormal chromosomal number in the developing embryos (Rho et al., 1998a; Liu and Yang, 1999). Therefore, 6-DMAP treatment has been delayed for 3 hours after activation with the calcium spike-inducing activator (ionomycin) to allow extrusion of the second polar body (Rho et al., 1998b).

1.3.2. Compromised Sperm Chromatin Remodeling

In bovine ICSI, remodeling of sperm chromatin was often compromised as the injected sperm heads either still kept its original shape or initially decondensed but never developed to paternal pronucleus (Li et al., 1999). To improve remodeling the sperm chromatin after ICSI, bull sperm have been treated with a disulphide bond-reducing agent, dithiothreitol (DTT) (Rho et al., 1998a; Ock et al., 2003; Galli et al., 2003; Rho et al., 2004). Bull sperm chromatin associated with cystein-rich type-I protamine, which is maximally cross-linked with disulfide bonds (Perreault et al., 1988a), are more stable than other species sperm chromatin associated with type-II protamine. The DTT treatment of bull spermatozoa was proven efficient to improve the pronucleus formation (Rho et al., 1998a; Ock et al., 2003) and to accelerate the kinetics of blastocyst formation (Galli et al., 2003). However, normal remodeling of bull sperm chromatin in bovine oocytes after IVF indicates that the compromised sperm chromatin remodeling after ICSI is probably due to isolation of the sperm chromatin from remodeling machinery in the ooplasm. Removing or extensive damaging the sperm plasma membrane immediately before ICSI by repeated freeze-thawing without cryoprotectant, scoring the tail against the base of the injection dish, or application of several piezo pulses to the mid-piece (Horiuchi et al., 2002; Galli et al., 2003), may accelerate the direct contact of sperm chromatin with intracellular remodeling machinery in the ooplasm and facilitate the interaction of the sperm-borne oocyte-activating factor (SOAF) with the ooplasm.

1.3.3. Technical Difficulties

Unlike mouse oocytes, bovine ooplasm contains lipid droplets at a very high concentration and the oolemma is highly elastic and tough so that blunt-ended injection pipette can be pushed deeply without rupture of the oolemma (nearly center of the oocyte). This characteristics results in a great difficulty at the time of ICSI, because the operator cannot confirm the rupture of the oolemma and injection of the spermatozoon. The problem of high elasticity and toughness of the bovine oolemma has been greatly overcome by application of piezo-ICSI (Katayose et al., 1999) where the piezo-electric effect is used to transmit a small crystal lattice distortion to the tip of a pipette, driving it forward in a precise and controlled manner. The piezo-actuated micromanipulation can result in non-lethal rupture of oolemma even with tips with a relatively large outer diameter (Yoshida and Perry, 2007). Centrifugation of bovine oocytes made it possible to visualize the tip of injection pipette (Tatham et al., 1996; Wei and Fukui, 2000), and facilitated the detection of oolemma rupture and the minimization of the volume of holding medium injected into the oocytes (Rho et al., 1998a; Wei and Fukui, 2000; Wei and Fukui, 2002). Although calves have been produced after injection of sperm head (Hamano et al., 1999), the common procedure for bovine ICSI includes injection of whole sperm as it is believed that sperm centrosome is essential for apposing the pronuclei after fertilization in this species (Navara et al., 1994; Shin and Kim, 2003). Partial removal of the bull sperm tail may improve the efficiency of ICSI through reduction of volume of the injected medium (Wei and Fukui, 2000; Wei and Fukui, 2002). Successful production of live offspring after ICSI in different species indicates that oocytes can decompose or eliminate the sperm component as plasma membrane and acrosomal contents which do not enter into ooplasm under physiological fertilization. However, it has been suggested that removal of the sperm cell membrane and acrosome immediately before ICSI, especially for animal species having large acrosome, may be preferable to activation of oocytes and embryonic development after ICSI (Morozumi and Yanagimachi, 2005; Morozumi et al., 2006).

2. Recent Progress: ICSI Versus IVF

2.1. DNA Demethylation in Pronuclear Zygotes

Epigenetic reprogramming in early preimplantation embryos, which refers to erasing and remodeling epigenetic marks, such as DNA methylation and/or histone phosphorylation, acetylation and methylation, is essential for differentiation and development. DNA methylation is one of the most-studied epigenetic mechanisms that can regulate the gene expression without changing the DNA consequences (Wu and Morris, 2001), and it is recognized as a chief contributor to the stability of gene expression state (Bird, 2002). While genomic methylation pattern is generally stable and heritable in differentiated somatic cells, mammalian genome undergoes a genome-wide methylation reprogramming in germ cells and preimplantation embryos (Reik et al., 2001; Li, 2002). In the early embryonic stage, the gametic methylation marks are erased (demethylation) and replaced with embryonic marks that are important for embryonic development and acquirement of toti- or pluripotency (Reik et al., 2001; Meehan, 2003). Then, the genome is subjected to de novo methylation process to establish the basic somatic bimodal methylation pattern at the time of implantation. The de novo methylation process commences at 8–16 cell stage in bovine embryos (Bourc'his et al., 2001) and in the inner cell mass (ICM) cells of mouse blastocysts (Santos et al., 2002). The reprogramming process organizes a fixed expression pattern in the genome by which tissue specific genes are globally repressed while housekeeping genes are active in all type of the cells.

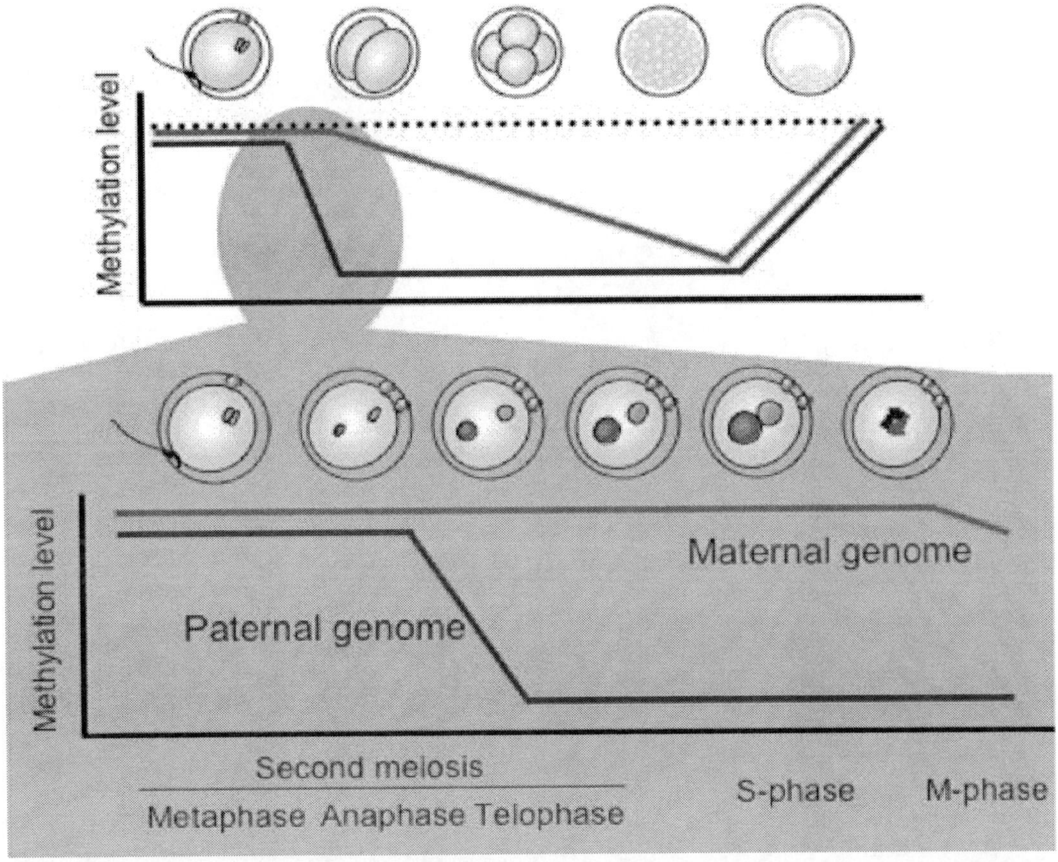

Figure 3. DNA demethylation during early embryonic development. Paternal genome undergoes replication-independent, genome-wide active demethylation while maternal genome maintains its methylation level until the beginning of mitotic division stage when both maternal and paternal genomes undergo replication-dependent, passive demethylation with each mitotic cycle. The extent of active demethylation in paternal genome varies from species to species.

From the recent researches on DNA methylation reprogramming, it was amazing that the demethylation dynamics of the paternal genome is different from that of the maternal genome (Figure 3). Evidences from pronuclear zygotes in some mammalian species indicate that paternal genome is subjected to replication-independent, genome-wide active demethylation during the first few hours after fertilization (Bourc'his et al., 2001; Santos et al., 2002). In contrary, maternal genome maintains its methylation level until the beginning of mitotic division stage when both maternal and paternal genomes undergo replication-dependent, passive demethylation with each mitotic cycle (Rougier et al., 1998). While the passive demethylation of the maternal genome may be due to the absence of methyltransferase maintenance enzyme (Dnmt1), many aspects relating to the active demethylation of paternal genome remain questionable (Wilkins, 2005). Although the active demethylation process of the sperm genome is considered to be a function of an ooplasmic factor(s), this process can be facilitated either by a sperm factor(s) or by male pronuclear chromatin composition (Beaujean et al., 2004).

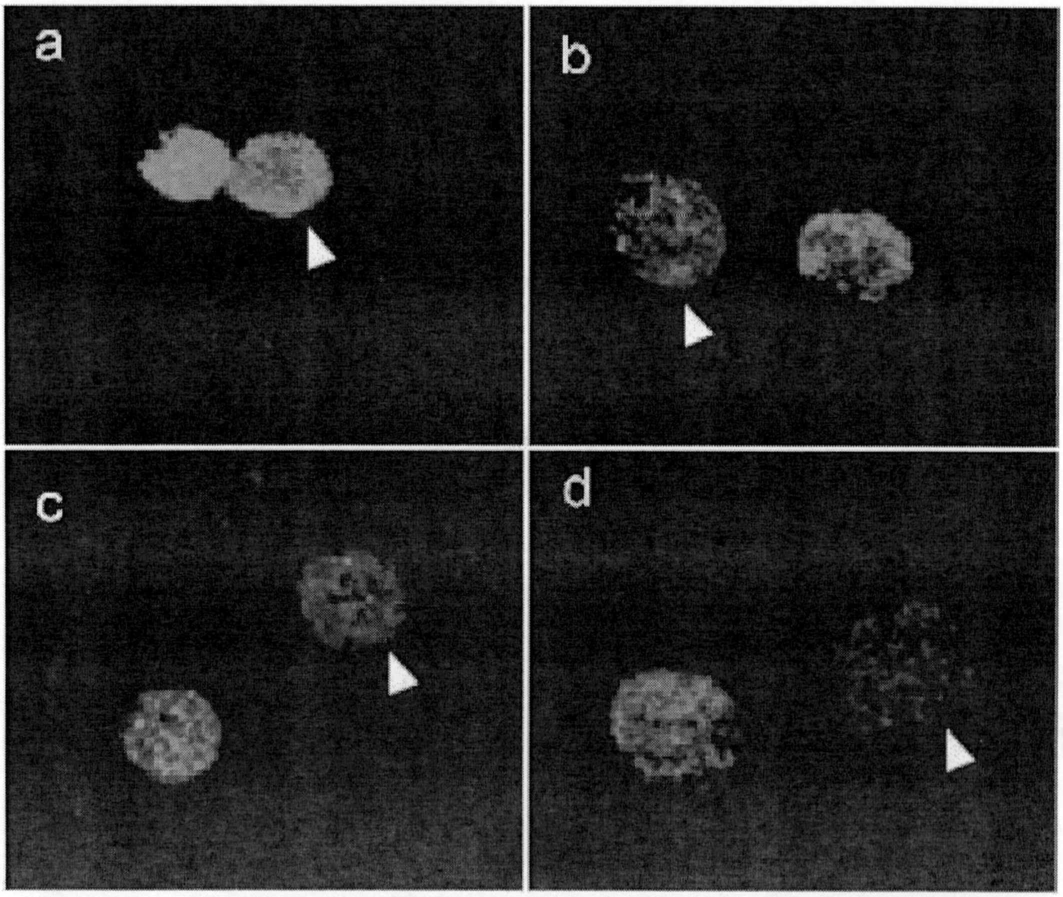

Figure 4. Pronuclear-stage bovine zygotes showing different levels of paternal genome methylation. Zygotes were treated with anti-5-methylcytosine (5-MeC) for analyzing methylated DNA level quantitatively. (a) RM=1.0; (b) RM=0.8; (c) RM=0.6; (d) RM=0.4. Arrows indicate male pronucleus.

The kinetics and the extent of active demethylation in pronuclear-stage zygotes, expressed as relative methylation of the paternal genome to the maternal counterpart (RM; Figure 4), are widely variable among different mammalian species with even conflicting results in some species. Such variability may indicate that the active demethylation of paternal genome is not obligate requirement for mammalian development; otherwise it seems that each species may have its own characteristic strategy required for the normal embryonic development. Although there is agreement that bovine paternal genomes undergo active demethylation (Bourc'his et al., 2001; Dean et al., 2001; Park et al., 2007), the extent of the demethylation process varies considerably, and the timing of this active demethylation remains unclear. Characterization of this strategy in bovine species would be helpful in understanding the biological significance of DNA methylation, including the mechanism by which normal embryonic development is regulated.

The IVF system is conventionally used to produce bovine embryos and offspring, and ICSI has been also resulted in successful production of live calves (Goto et al., 1990; Hamano et al., 1999). However, epigenetic defects have been found in human babies derived from ICSI (Cox et al., 2002; Nikolettos et al., 2006). We investigated the dynamics of the active methylation process of the paternal genome in pronuclear-stage bovine zygotes produced by ICSI and IVF (Abdalla et al., 2009a). Immunostaining protocol against 5-methylcytosine was used for quantitative analysis of the genome-wide demethylation dynamics in pronuclear bovine zygotes, as reported previously (Dean et al., 2001; Park et al., 2007). The demethylation dynamics of the pronuclear-stage IVF-derived zygotes harvested at 8, 10, 14 and 18 hours post-insemination (hpi), and of the ICSI-derived zygotes harvested at 6 and 12 hpi are shown in Table 2. Since it takes about 2 hours until spermatozoa can penetrate into the oocytes in bovine IVF system, ICSI zygotes at 6 and 12 hpi were considered developmentally comparable with IVF zygotes at 8 and 14 hpi. In IVF-derived zygotes, the overall average of the RM significantly decreased from 0.92 at 8 hpi to 0.69 at 10 hpi without any additional decrease at 14 and 18 hpi. This was accompanied with higher proportions of zygotes showing RM<0.6 at 10, 14 and 18 hpi, compared to the proportion at 8 hpi. Moreover, the RM values in some zygotes were less than 0.4. The overall averages of the RM in ICSI-derived zygotes (0.79 at 6 hpi and 0.66 at 12 hpi) were similar to those in the corresponding IVF-derived zygotes (8 and 14 hpi), but higher proportion of the 6 hpi zygotes showed RM<0.6 compared to the 8 hpi IVF-derived zygotes. Moreover, the proportion of zygotes showing RM<0.6 did not increase after prolonged culture in the ICSI-derived zygotes (37.8 versus 39.4% for 6 versus 12 hpi) but increased in the IVF-derived zygotes (3.7 versus 40.6% for 8 versus 14 hpi). Thus, paternal genome rapidly demethylated within 10 hours after IVF and 6 hours after ICSI. The demethylation extent in pronuclear zygotes was moderate with 0.4≤RM<0.6.

Park et al. (2007) reported that the overall averages of the RM in the IVF-derived bovine zygotes decreased from 0.84±0.13 at 10 hpi to 0.51±0.19 at 20 hpi. This coincides with the time-dependent, significant reduction of methylation status of the paternal genome in the IVF-derived bovine zygotes observed in our study (from 8 to 18 hpi; Abdalla et al., 2009a). However, initiation and completion of demethylation of the bovine paternal genome occurred very early without any further reduction after a prolonged culture period. The different finding regarding the methylation status of the paternal genome at 10 hpi between our study and that of Park et al. (2007) may be due to the different systems employed for in vitro production of bovine zygotes (*e.g.*, use of oocytes with or without cumulus cells during insemination, and different co-incubation periods). The timing of paternal genome demethylation in bovine zygotes (8-10 hpi) was comparatively earlier than the onset time of DNA replication, which occurs as late as 17 hpi (Comizzoli et al., 2000). Remethylation of the paternal genome after the demethylation process, which has been reported to occur in bovine zygotes at 25 hpi (Park et al., 2007), was not observed in our study. As to the demethylation dynamics in ICSI-derived zygotes, there were no significant differences in the overall average of RM and the proportions of zygotes showing RM<0.6 between 6 and 12 hpi zygotes. Contrastly, similar dynamics of paternal genome demethylation between ICSI- and IVF-derived zygotes has been reported in mouse (Fulka and Fulka, 2006). This difference may be due to that the 6 hpi zygotes with a narrow fertilization window (15 min) are older than the 8 hpi zygotes a with wide fertilization window (2 hours) and/or that the ICSI protocol using a piezo-driven pipette contains a factor(s) hastening the demethylation process. The pronuclear size of the ICSI-derived zygotes at 6 hpi was similar to that of the IVF-derived zygotes at 8 hpi, but the size of the male pronucleus was not correlated with the individual RM value at any time points in all experimental groups. This suggests that the process of the paternal genome demethylation is independent from the process of chromatin decondensation (Santos et al., 2002).

Table 2. Dynamics of paternal DNA demethylation in IVF- and ICSI-derived bovine zygotes

Age of zygotes	No.(%) of oocytes Inseminated	Penetrated	2PN	No.(%) of zygotes Analyzed	RM<0.6	0.6≤RM≤1.0	RM>1.0	Mean RM ±SEM
IVF-derived zygotes								
8 hpi	76	65 (85.5)	31 (40.8)^{c}	27	1 (3.7)^{b}	19 (70.4)^{a}	7 (25.9)^{a}	0.92±0.04^{a}
10 hpi	55	48 (87.3)	35 (63.6)^{ab}	33	15 (45.5)^{a}	14 (42.4)^{b}	4 (12.1)^{ab}	0.69±0.06^{b}
14 hpi	60	52 (86.7)	33 (55.0)^{b}	32	12 (37.5)^{a}	18 (56.2)^{ab}	2 (6.3)^{b}	0.67±0.04^{b}
18 hpi	56	53 (94.6)	40 (71.4)^{a}	34	13 (38.2)^{a}	17 (50.0)^{ab}	4 (11.8)^{ab}	0.64±0.04^{b}
ICSI-derived zygotes								
6 hpi	144	---	43 (29.9)^{ab}	37	14 (37.8)^{a}	17 (45.9)^{ab}	6 (16.2)^{ab}	0.79±0.07^{a}
12 hpi	74	---	36 (48.6)^{a}	33	13 (39.4)^{a}	18 (54.5)^{ab}	3 (6.1)^{b}	0.66±0.05^{b}

Values with different superscripts within the same columns are significantly different (P<0.05).
Abbreviations; hpi: hours post-insemination, 2PN: two pronuclei, RM: relative methylation.
Data are from Abdalla et al. (2009a).

2.2. Yield And Quality of Day 7-8 Blastocysts

In most of mammalian species, the ovulated oocytes or in-vitro matured oocytes are arrested at the M-II. This arrest is maintained by high level of MPF composed of a catalytic cyclin-dependent kinase-1 (Cdk1/cdc2) and a regulatory subunit (cyclin-B) (Gautier et al., 1990). High activity of the MPF is controlled by some cytostatic factor(s) (CSF) which either increases the synthesis of cyclin B or inhibits its lysis mechanism. Metaphase-anaphase transition occurs through polyubiquitination of cyclin B by anaphase-promoting complex / cyclosome (APC/C) that initiates immediate proteolysis of the cyclin B and subsequently results in decrease of the MPF activity (Huo et al., 2004; Jones, 2005; Brunet and Maro, 2005). The resumption of meiosis can be triggered by sperm penetration or parthenogenetical activation treatment (Liu and Yang, 1999; Malcuit et al., 2006a). At fertilization, the sperm evoke several increases in the intracellular calcium concentration (calcium oscillations), which may be responsible for initiation and completion of many post-fertilization events, as cortical granule exocytosis (McAvey et al., 2002), resumption of meiosis, pronucleus formation, recruitment of maternal mRNAs, and initiation of mitotic division (Scultze and Kopf, 1995; Ducibella et al., 2002).

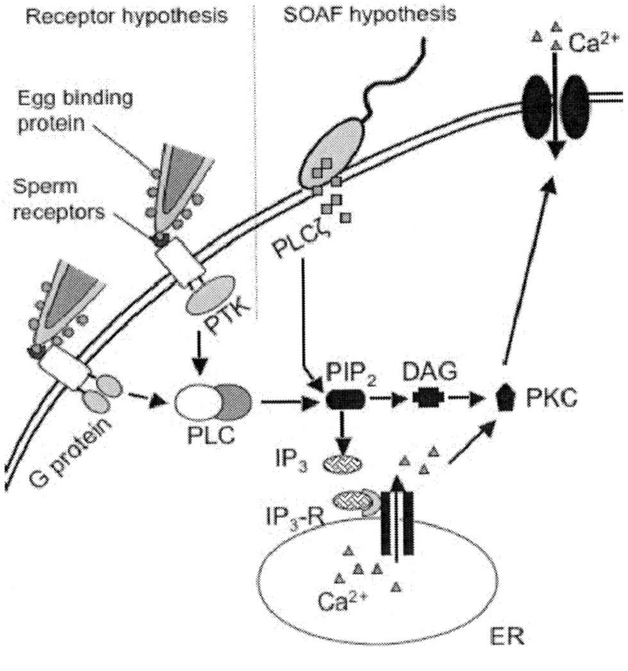

Figure 5. Possible mechanisms for occurrence of intracellular calcium oscillations induced by spermatozoa. Receptor hypothesis with the receptor / GTP binding protein (G protein) / phosphoinositol pathway, or the receptor / protein tyrosine kinase (PTK) / PI pathway is presented. Binding of the sperm with receptor in the oocyte membrane activates a phosphoinositide-specific phospholipase-C (PLC) and in turn stimulates the PI pathway, resulting in the production of inositol-1,4,5-triphosphate (IP3) and 1,2-diacyl glycerol (DAG) from phosphatidylinositol-4,5-bisphosphate (PIP2). Alternatively, SOAF hypothesis is presented. The SOAF, thought to be PLCζ, is introduced into oocytes and stimulates the PI pathway. In all cases, the IP3 binds to its receptor (IP3-R) present in the endoplasmic reticulum (ER, the main Ca^{2+} store in the cell) and gating the receptors to release the Ca^{2+} store into the ooplasm. The DAG with the intracellular calcium activates protein kinase C which translocates to the plasma membrane and regulates Ca^{2+} influx to refill the intracellular stores.

The calcium oscillations even have a great impact on the developmental performance (Ozil and Huneau, 2001). Several theories that explain the mechanism by which the calcium oscillations occur (Malcuit et al., 2006a; Miyazaki and Ito, 2006) are presented in Figure 5. It has been established in all species that the calcium oscillations mainly occur through activation of phosphoinositide pathway (Fissore et al., 1995; Wu et al., 2001; Malciute et al.,

2005) without eliminating the possible role of other receptors as ryanodine receptors (Wu et al., 1997). Although the nature of sperm component responsible for induction of oocyte activation is still controversial, a possible candidate of the SOAF is phospholipase C-zeta (PLCζ) or substance that activates the upstream of egg PLCζ (Wu et al., 2001; Williams, 2002; Bedford et al., 2006). The intracellular calcium increases induce a calcium-dependent inactivation of MPF through degradation of its regulatory subunit (cyclin-B) (Lorca et al., 1993), followed by inactivation of MAPK (mitogen-activated protein kinase) which is associated with pronuclear development (Liu and Yang, 1999). The degree of oocyte activation has been found to be affected by the number of calcium oscillations and the duration of the sustained calcium signals (Ducibella et al., 2002; Ozil et al., 2005). In bovine IVF, the calcium oscillations begin 1 min after sperm-egg contact and last for several hours at a constant interval (20 min) until pronuclear migration and nuclear envelop breakdown (Nakada et al., 1995, 1998). This oscillation pattern may be sufficient for initiation and completion of calcium-dependent, post-fertilization events.

Prior to pronuclear formation, remodeling of sperm chromatin occurs. After incorporation of the sperm heads into ooplasm, the highly condensed and transcriptionally inert chromatin of the spermatozoa is initially dispersed, then transitionally recondenses, and finally extensively decondenses into transcriptionally competent chromatin in the paternal pronucleus (Mclay and Clarke, 2003). The oocytes acquire the ability to remodel the sperm chromatin during its maturation (Mclay and Clarke, 1997). The remodeling ability of oocytes is directly related to the ooplasmic content of glutathione, an endogenous reducing agent that protects cells from oxidation stresses and exerts a number of important roles in cellular metabolism (Sutovsky and Schatten, 1997). The pool of glutathione seems to assure the reduction of disulfide bonds in the sperm nucleus and thus promotes its decondensation into the paternal pronucleus (Perreault et al., 1988b). Chemical inhibition of the disulphide bond-reducing activity of the oocytes disturbed the decondensation of injected sperm nuclei (Perreault et al., 1984).

Developmental potential of ICSI oocytes into blastocysts in vitro is still low, probably due to the inability of the mechanical stimulation and/or the injected spermatozoon itself to induce proper oocyte activation after ICSI. Therefore, we have directly compared several protocols for inducing activation in bovine ICSI oocytes (Adballa et al., 2009b). As shown in Figure 6, the cleavage rates of ICSI oocytes treated with ionomycin plus ethanol or CHX (69-78%) were similar to that after IVF (86%) and higher than that of non-treated oocytes (39%). However, treating the oocytes with ethanol alone, ionomycin alone or ionomycin plus 6-DMAP did not improve the cleavage rate (45-61%). Although the proportions of the cleaved zygotes developed into blastocysts until Day-8 were statistically similar among all groups (19-43%), these proportions were obviously lower in ionomycin alone, ionomycin + CHX or ionomycin + 6-DMAP groups (19, 24 or 21%, respectively) than in ionomycin + ethanol groups and IVF group (38-43% and 46%, respectively). Moreover, ionomycin plus ethanol treatment significantly improved the proportions of ICSI oocytes developing into blastocysts until Day-8 (29-30%) compared to non-treated oocytes (12%). These improved yields were comparable with that after IVF (40%). Thus, the new activation regimen composed from two triggers for single calcium increase (5 μM ionomycin for 5 min immediately after ICSI plus 7% ethanol for 5 min 4 hours after ICSI) without using either protein synthesis or protein phosphorylation inhibitors was applicable to the ICSI oocytes.

Our blastocyst yield in non-treated group (12%) is higher than those (0-8%) reported previously by several laboratories (Rho et al., 1998a; Keskintepe and Brackett, 2000; Emuta and Horiuchi, 2001; Horiuchi et al., 2002; Ock et al., 2003; Fujinami et al., 2004; Oikawa et al., 2005), but comparable to or even lower than those (15-23%) in other reports (Wei and Fukui, 2002; Galli et al., 2003).

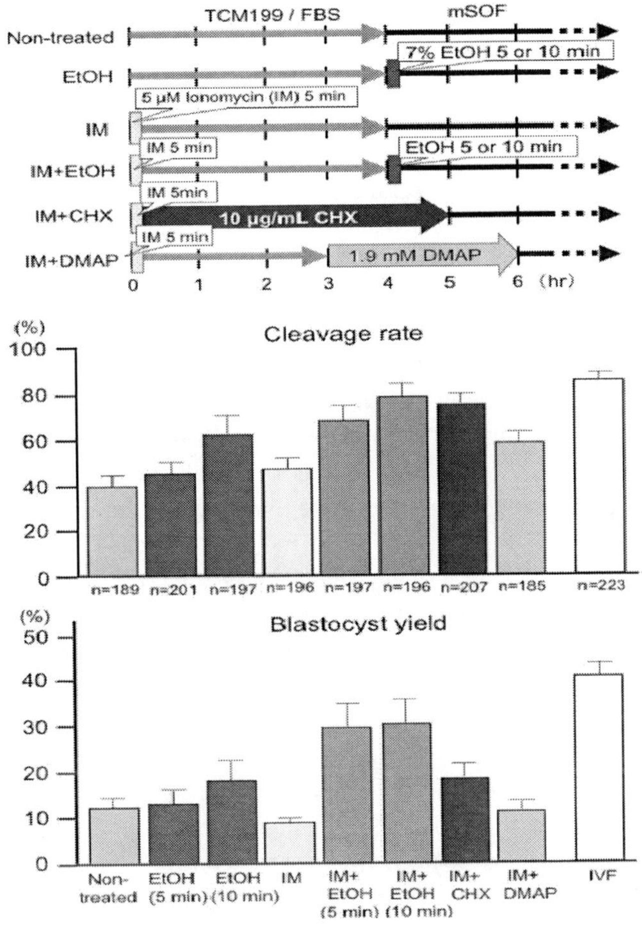

Figure 6. In vitro development of bovine ICSI oocytes after different activation treatments. Non-centrifuged oocytes injected with DTT-treated sperm were allocated to one of the following treatments: (1) Non-treated; Injected oocytes were incubated in TCM-199/FBS medium at 38.5 °C under 5% CO_2 in air for 4 hours. (2) Ethanol (EtOH) alone; Injected oocytes were incubated for 4 hours as described above, and then treated with 7% EtOH in TCM-199 supplemented with 1 mg/mL PVP-40 for 5 or 10 min. (3) Ionomycin (IM) alone; Injected oocytes were treated with 5 mM IM in a Ca^{2+}- and Mg^{+2}-free PBS for 5 min immediately after ICSI. (4) IM + EtOH; Injected oocytes were first treated with IM immediately after ICSI as described above, and incubated in the TCM-199/FBS medium for 4 hours. Next, the oocytes were treated with 7% EtOH for 5 or 10 min, as described above. (5) IM + CHX; Injected oocytes were first treated with IM immediately after ICSI as described above, and followed by incubation in culture medium containing 10 μg/mL CHX for 5 hours. (6) IM + 6-DMAP; Injected oocytes were first treated with IM immediately after ICSI as described above, and incubated in the TCM-199/FBS medium for 3 hours. Next, the oocytes were incubated in culture medium containing 1.9 mM 6-DMAP for an additional 3 hours. Cleavage (Day-2) and development into blastocysts (Day-7 and -8) of IVF-derived zygotes are also shown for direct comparison. Data are from Abdalla et al. (2009b).

However, blastocysts/ cleavage rate in our study (30%) is comparable to that reported by Wei and Fukui (2002) (32%) which indicates that a failure in the early post-fertilization events -from fertilization until cleavage- is the main determiner to the successful development after bovine ICSI. Application of additional activation stimuli to the bovine ICSI oocytes have been considered important for decondensation of sperm heads, pronuclear formation, cleavage and embryonic development (Rho et al., 1998a). Since induction of abnormally high frequent and/or prolonged calcium elevation may trigger premature termination of embryonic development (Gordo et al., 2000), the additional activation stimuli better to mimic the mechanism induced during normal fertilization without affecting other oocytes metabolic pathway. Ooplasmic injection of a promising SOAF candidate, PLCζ or its cRNA (Ross et al., 2008) was applied as a more physiological approach, but complicated steps required for isolation of this substance or preparation of its cRNA as well as difficulty to control the injected volumes make this method far from practical.

A simplest regimen proved effective to improve blastocyst production after bovine ICSI, using only a trigger for inducing a single calcium increase in oocytes, was to treat the oocytes 4 hours after ICSI with 7% ethanol solution for 5 min (Emuta and Horiuchi, 2001; Horiuchi et al., 2002; Fujinami et al., 2004; Oikawa et al., 2005). Our blastocyst yield by this protocol (13%) was comparable to those reported by some previous literatures (14-21%) (Emuta and Horiuchi, 2001; Horiuchi et al., 2002; Fujinami et al., 2004) but lower than that reported by Oikawa et al. (2005) (29%). This protocol was originally applied to the ICSI oocytes that extruded the second polar body; in another word, the oocytes that received activation stimuli -from the sperm- enough for the resumption of meiosis. Fujinami et al. (2004) reported that bovine oocytes showed re-elevation of MPF at 6 hours after sperm injection, and that treating those oocytes with ethanol prevents this re-elevation. Our unsatisfactory blastocyst yield by this protocol was probably due to the lower proportion of ICSI oocytes extruding the second polar body at the time of ethanol activation (45-46%) compared to that (60-70%) reported by Horiuchi et al. (2002). In order to increase the ICSI oocytes that extruded the second polar body at the time of ethanol treatment, oocytes were treated with 5 μM ionomycin immediately after ICSI. This attempt significantly improved the Day 7-8 blastocyst yields (29-30% of overall oocytes) without significant improvement in the blastocyst yield per cleaved zygote (38-43% versus 30% in non-treated control). This suggests that, in bovine ICSI, the early post-fertilization events from fertilization up to the first cleavage have a great impact on the successful development of the embryos.

Another activation regimen proved effective to improve blastocyst yield after bovine ICSI is to combine ionomycin with 6-DMAP (Rho et al., 1998a; Ock et al., 2003; Oikawa et al., 2005). In our study, neither the cleavage rate nor the blastocyst yield was improved regardless of the improved proportion of the second polar body extrusion after this treatment. This result was contradictory to some previous reports (Rho et al., 1998a; Ock et al., 2003; Oikawa et al., 2005) but in agreement with the report by Keskintepe et al. (2002). Using CHX instead of 6-DMAP improved the cleavage rate but not the blastocyst yield, which is in agreement with the report by Galli et al. (2003). Moreover, both activation regimens (ionomycin plus CHX or 6-DMAP) resulted in obviously low blastocyst yield per cleaved zygote (21-23%). Thus, the significantly lower blastocyst yields from the ICSI oocytes treated with ionomycin plus CHX or 6-DMAP may be reflected by the adverse effects of the inhibitors employed here (CHX and 6-DMAP) on the activity of other kinases or the synthesis of the other proteins involved in other cell functions rather than regulation of cell cycle (Soloy et al., 1997). Using more specific kinase inhibitors for cell cycle regulation (Perecin et al., 2007) may avoid such side effects of CHX or 6-DMAP.

One disadvantage of the application of exogenous activation is to increase the possibility of the parthenogenetic development (Li et al., 1999). In our study (Abdalla et al., 2009b), only a few blastocysts (1-2%) were obtained during 8-days culture after chemical or physical parthenogenetic treatments. In addition, we have a similar result after parthenogenetic activation of sham-injected oocytes with ionomycin and ethanol. Chemicals such as ethanol, ionomycin or calcium ionophore combined with or without CHX were not sufficient to induce parthenogenetic development in bovine oocytes (Winger et al., 1997; Liu et al., 1998). Induction of diploidization by combining the calcium oscillation-inducing activators with cytochalasin or 6-DMAP was necessary to improve the parthenogenetic development of bovine oocytes (Liu et al., 1998; Rho et al., 1998b; Méo et al., 2004). This may explain the complete failure or very low parthenogenetic developmental rate after different activation protocols in our study. However, relatively high proportions of parthenogenetic development have been reported after activation of sham-injected bovine oocytes with calcium oscillations-inducible chemicals without diploidization (Rho et al., 1998a; Ock et al., 2003; Oikawa et al., 2005).

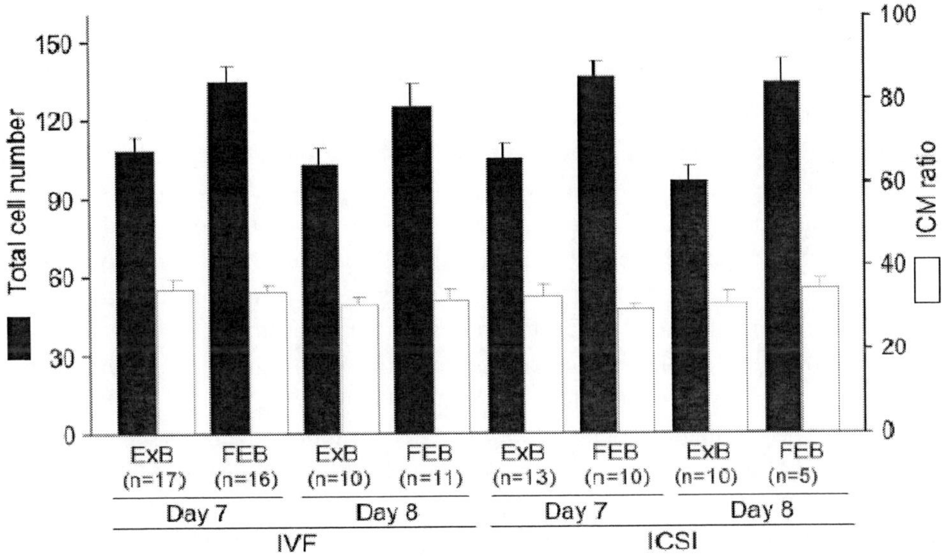

Figure 7. Quality analysis of IVF- and ICSI-derived bovine blastocysts by differential staining for ICM/TE cells. ExB: Expanding blastocysts, FEB: Fully-expanded blastocysts. Mean number or ratio ± S.E.M. Data are from Abdalla et al. (2010).

Undoubtedly, the most precise evidence for the quality of the in-vitro produced bovine embryos is their ability to develop into full-term calves after transfer to recipient animals. However, the total cell number of the blastocysts, the ratio of ICM cells, as well as the developmental kinetics until blastocoele formation are often used as alternative parameters to assess the quality of the blastocysts (Van Soom et al., 1997). Quality analysis of Day-7 expanding blastocysts by differential cell counting (Abdalla et al., 2009b) indicated that there were no significant differences in the total cell number or the ratio of the ICM cells among ICSI derived-blastocysts derived from non-treated oocytes (128 cells and 37%, respectively), those derived after different activation treatments (108-135 cells and 30-39%, respectively) and those derived after IVF (121 cells and 34%, respectively). None of the regimens had any adverse effect on the quality of the blastocysts regarding the total cell number or the proportion of the ICM cells. In addition, ICSI-derived as well as IVF-derived blastocysts harvested on Day-7 or -8 were classified into one of two developmental stages; fully-expanded blastocysts that were ≥200 μm in diameter, or expanding blastocysts that were 140 to 199 μm in diameter (Abdalla et al., 2010). Out of 1,384 IVF-derived zygotes cultured, 1,101 (80%) cleaved on Day-2, and 406 (29%) and 156 (11%) developed to expanding or fully-expanded blastocysts on Day-7 and -8, respectively. In addition, out of 1,061 ICSI-derived zygotes cultured, 798 (68%) cleaved on Day-2, and 155 (15%) and 87 (8%) developed to expanding or fully-expanded blastocysts on Day-7 and -8. The ICM cell ratio (31- 35%) was not affected by the method of embryo production (IVF versus ICSI), the day of blastocyst harvest (Day-7 versus Day-8), or developmental stage (expanding versus fully-expanded), as shown in Figure 7. Fully-expanded blastocysts tended to have higher total cell number (ranged from 125 to 136 cells) than expanding blastocysts (ranged from 96 to 108 cells), regardless of the method of embryo production or day of blastocyst harvest.

2.3. Cryotolerance of Expanding and Fully-Expanded Blastocysts

Sensitivity of the bovine embryos to cryopreservation is affected by many factors including the method of embryo production (in vivo- versus in vitro-derived), the embryo quality and the developmental age and stage. While numerous studies indicated that the in vitro-produced embryos, mainly IVF-derived zygotes, have lower cryotolerance than the in vivo-derived counterparts (Massip et al., 1995), the culture conditions used for the IVF-derived presumptive zygotes have been found to greatly influence the cryotolerance of these embryos (Mucci et al., 2006; Shirazi et al., 2009). As to the developmental age, the faster-developing IVF-derived bovine blastocysts (harvested 7 days after insemination; Day-7) were reported to be more tolerable to the cryopreservation than the slower-developing ones (harvested 8 days after insemination; Day-8) (Han et al., 1994; Saha et al., 1996). Among the blastocysts developed in the same day, embryos reaching more advanced stage or larger size were found to have higher ability to survive the cryopreservation procedures (Han et al., 1994; Dinnyés et al., 1999).

The main cryoinjury during the freezing process is resulted from formation of the intracellular ice crystals. Vitrification, which involves an extreme increase in the viscosity of the cryoprotective solution and completely eliminates the ice crystal formation, has become a promising alternative to the freezing to improve the cryotolerance of the IVF-derived embryos (Mucci et al., 2006; Nedambale et al., 2004). The vitrification procedure requires utilization of extremely high concentration of the cryoprotectants and achieving extremely high cooling and warming rate. The utilization of the cryoprotectants in a high concentration may be toxic or result in osmotic stress to the embryos (Liebermann et al., 2002). The only way to induce the vitrification using lower concentration of the cryoprotectants is to increase the cooling rate. Application of different cryodevices that reduce the volume of vitrification solution (minimum volume cooling: MVC) and/or decreasing the temperature of the liquid nitrogen (N_2 slush) has been attempted to increase the cooling rate (Vajta and Kuwayama M, 2006). Cryotop technology, an advanced version of the MVC procedure, has been originally developed for cryopreservation of human oocytes and embryos (Kuwayama and Kato, 2000), and successfully applied to vitrify oocytes from different species (Liu et al., 2008; Morató et al., 2008), IVF-derived embryos (Kelly et al., 2004; De Rosa et al., 2007) and reconstructed embryos with somatic cell nuclei (Laowtammathron et al., 2005; Du et al., 2007).

There is only one publication regarding cryopreservation of ICSI-derived bovine embryos (Keskintepe and Brackett, 2000), which showed that 75% (12/16) of Day-7 expanded blastocysts and 88% (14/16) of Day-8 hatched blastocysts survived the conventional two-step freezing. These cryosurvival rates in ICSI-derived embryos seemed to be comparable with those in IVF-derived counterparts. However, the ability of ICSI-derived bovine embryos to survive vitrification has not been reported yet. Therefore, we investigated the effects of developmental stage (fully-expanded or expanding blastocysts) and/or age (Day-7 or -8) on the survival of ICSI-derived versus IVF-derived bovine blastocysts after vitrification (Abdalla et al., 2010). Blastocysts were cryopreserved by the MVC-Cryotop vitrification procedure, and the post-warming survival was assessed by their ability to reexpand during 24 hours of in vitro culture (Figure 8). The post-warming survival rates of IVF-derived blastocysts (84 to 89%) were not affected by the developmental stage or age, as shown in Table 3. Conversely in the ICSI group, the ability of fully-expanded Day-7 or -8 ICSI-derived blastocysts to survive the vitrification procedures tended to be higher than that of the expanding-stage counterparts, and the difference reached a significant level when the data were pooled across the day of blastocyst harvest (80 versus 61%). The cryosurvival of the IVF-derived expanding blastocysts were significantly higher than that of the ICSI-derived counterparts, regardless of the day of blastocyst harvest. Due to these differences, the overall cryosurvival of ICSI-derived blastocysts was significantly lower than that of IVF-derived counterparts (86 versus 69%). Thus, the ICSI-derived fully-expanded (≥200 μm in diameter) bovine blastocysts have similar ability to survive MVC-Cryotop vitrification to the IVF-derived counterparts. Since ICSI-derived, but not IVF-derived, expanding blastocysts were slightly sensitive to the vitrification procedure; it is recommended to continue the *in vitro* culture of the ICSI-derived embryos until reaching fully-expanded stage before cryopreservation.

Table 3. In vitro survival of IVF- and ICSI-derived bovine blastocysts after vitrification: Effect of developmental stage and embryonic age

Origin	Developmental stage	Embryonic age Day-7	Day-8	Subtotal
IVF	Fully-expanded	58 / 66 (88)^{x}	25 / 28 (89)^{x}	183 / 194 (88)^{xx}
	Expanded	63 / 74 (85)^{x}	32 / 38 (84)^{x}	195 / 112 (85)^{xx}
	Subtotal	121 / 140 (86)^{x}	57 / 66 (86)^{x}	178 / 206 (86)^{xx}
ICSI	Fully-expanded	25 / 30 (83)^{x}	11 / 15 (73)^{x}	136 / 145 (80)^{ax}
	Expanding	30 / 45 (67)^{y}	18 / 17 (47)^{y}	138 / 162 (61)^{by}
	Subtota	55 / 75 (73)^{y}	19 / 32 (59)^{y}	174 / 107 (69)^{yx}

No. of re-expanded embryos / No. of vitrified-warmed embryos (%).
a vs b: Significantly different between two developmental stages within IVF or ICSI group.
x vs y: Significantly different between IVF and ICSI groups.
Data are from Abdalla et al. (2010).

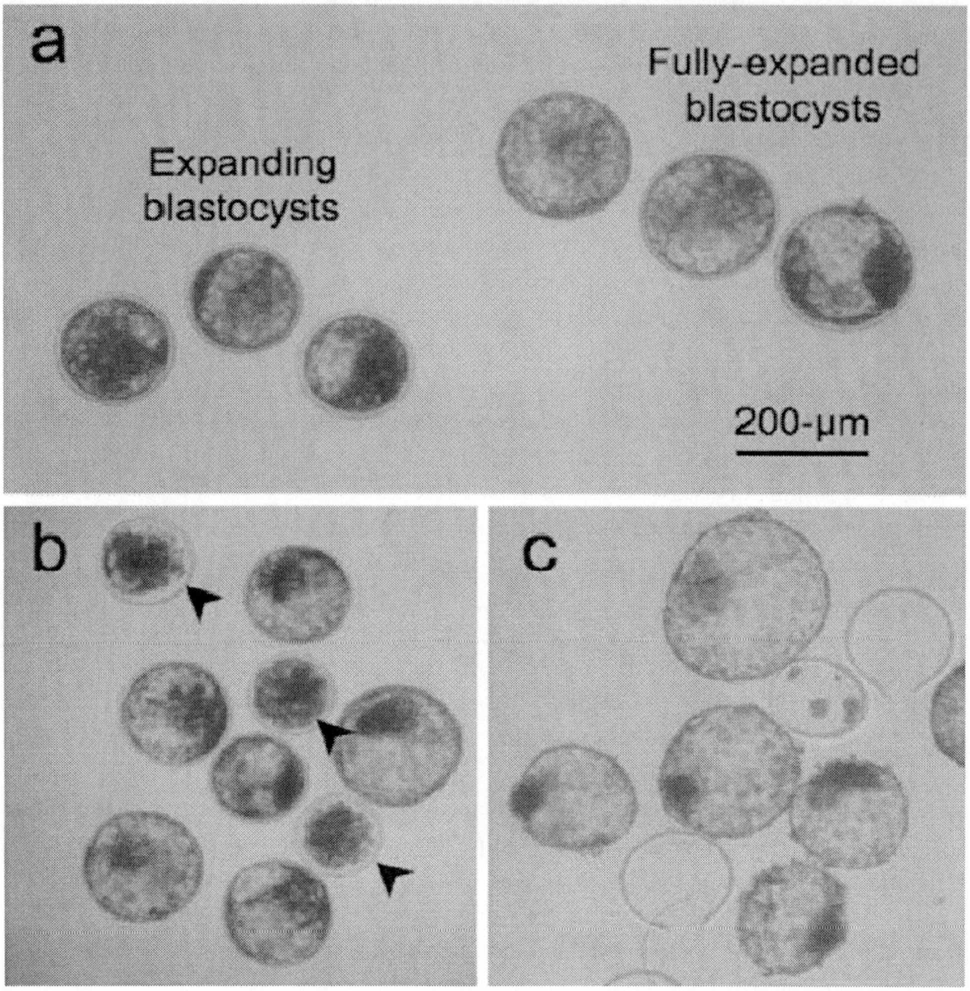

Figure 8. Morphology of *in vitro*-produced bovine blastocysts. (a) Fully-expanded blastocysts (≥ 200-µm in diameter) and expanding blastocysts (140-µm ≤ diameter < 200-µm). (b) Vitrified-warmed blastocysts after 24 hours of culture. Re-expanded blastocysts were judged as surviving, while embryos failed to re-expand (arrow heads) were considered as degenerated. (c) Hatched blastocysts after 72 hours of post-warm culture.

Differential cell staining for the fresh blastocysts indicated that ICSI-derived expanding blastocysts have comparable quality assessed by the total cell number and the ICM ratio to the IVF-derived counterparts (Figure 7), therefore the higher sensitivity of ICSI-derived expanding blastocysts to the MVC vitrification would be difficult to be explained by the difference in embryo quality before vitrification. The relationship between the size of blastocysts and their cryotolerance has been investigated and the results showed that the larger blastocysts are more tolerable to cryopreservation than the smaller ones (Dinnyés et al., 1996; George et al., 2008), with one exceptional report (Shirazi et al., 2009). It has been reported that tolerance to vitrification of IVF-derived bovine blastocysts was improved after their sizes reached 150-160 µm in diameter (Dinnyés et al., 1996; Dinnyés et al., 1999; George et al., 2008). The difference between the cryotolerance of the IVF- and ICSI-derived expanding blastocysts may be due to the fact that the size of the ICSI-derived expanding blastocysts was comparatively smaller than the IVF-derived ones, even though the mean total cell number was comparable.

There is also a general agreement that the faster-developing bovine embryos are more likely to survive the cryopreservation process (Han et al., 1994; Saha et al., 1996; Dinnyés et al., 1999). Therefore, most of the reports regarding embryo cryopreservation handled the blastocysts harvested on Day-7 either all or after additional morphological selection. Our cryosurvival rate of Day-7 IVF-derived blastocysts achieved using the Cryotop (86%; Abdalla et al., 2010) was slightly lower than 94% survival reported using the same cryodevice (Kelly et al., 2004), and was comparable to or even higher than those achieved using other cryodevices for MVC vitrification such as open-pulled straws (OPS; 89 to 97%; Vajta et al., 1999) and electron microscope grids (58-98%; Park et al., 1999). Moreover, our study showed that the Day-8 blastocysts have similar survivability to the Day-7 counterparts either in IVF- or ICSI-derived zygotes. Dinnyés et al. (1996) reported a reasonable cryosurvival rate from IVF-derived Day 8 bovine embryos at the fully-expanded and hatched blastocyst stages (<90%); however, those embryos were produced by prolonged culture of Day-7 blastocysts.

Conclusion

The ICSI technique has been used not only as a research tool for understanding fundamental aspects of gamete interaction during fertilization, but also as a practical alternative to conventional IVF in rescuing severe male infertility. In bovine, the ICSI technique can be applied to achieve the best utilization of genetically superior bulls characterized by low sperm concentration, low motility in their ejaculate or poor reaction with the in vitro capacitation process required for IVF protocol. Therefore, abilities of bovine embryos derived from ICSI were compared to those from IVF for the following categories. [1] Active DNA demethylation: Paternal genome rapidly demethylated within 10 hours after IVF and 6 hours after ICSI. The demethylation extent in pronuclear zygotes was moderate with $0.4 \leq RM < 0.6$. [2] Blastocyst yield: An activation regimen composed from two triggers for single calcium increase (5 μM ionomycin for 5 min immediately after ICSI plus 7% ethanol for 5 min 4 hours after ICSI) was found applicable to the ICSI oocytes, with a 30% yield comparable with 40% in IVF group. [3] Cryotolerance: The proportion of fully-expanded blastocysts that survived MVC-Cryotop vitrification procedure was similar for ICSI- and IVF-derived blastocysts (73-83% and 88-89%, respectively). For smaller ICSI-derived, but not for IVF-derived, blastocysts, further culture until reaching the expanded stage before vitrification is recommended.

References

Abdalla, H., Hirabayashi, M. and Hochi, S. (2009a) Demethylation dynamics of the paternal genome in pronuclear-stage bovine zygotes produced by in vitro fertilization and ooplasmic injection of freeze-thawed or freeze-dried spermatozoa. *J. Reprod. Dev.*, 55, 433–439.

Abdalla, H., Shimoda, M., Hara, H., Morita, H., Kuwayama, M., Hirabayashi, M. and Hochi, S. (2010) Vitrification of ICSI- and IVF-derived bovine blastocysts by minimum volume cooling procedure: effect of developmental stage and age. *Theriogenology,* 74, 1028–1035.

Abdalla, H., Shimoda, M., Hirabayashi, M. and Hochi, S. (2009b) A combined treatment of ionomycin with ethanol improves blastocyst development of bovine oocytes harvested from stored ovaries and microinjected with spermatozoa. *Theriogenology*, 72, 453–460.

Barnes, F.L. and First, N.L. (1991) Embryonic transcription in in vitro cultured bovine embryos. *Mol. Reprod. Dev*., 29, 117–123.

Bavister, B.D. (1995) Culture of preimplantation embryos: facts and artifacts. *Hum. Reprod. Update*, 1, 91–148.

Beaujean, N., Taylor, J.E., McGarry, M., Gardner, J.O., Wilmut, I., Loi, P., Ptak, G., Galli, C., Lazzari, G., Bird, A., Young, L.E. and Meehan, R.R. (2004) The effect of interspecific oocytes on demethylation of sperm DNA. *Proc. Natl. Acad. Sci. USA*, 101, 7636–7640.

Bird, A. (2002) DNA methylation patterns and epigenetic memory. *Genes Dev*., 16, 6–21.

Bourc'his, D., Le Bourhis, D., Patin, D., Niveleau, A., Comizzoli, P., Renard, J.P. and Viegas-Péquignot, E. (2001) Delayed and incomplete reprogramming of chromosome methylation patterns in bovine cloned embryos. *Curr. Biol*., 11, 1542–1546.

Brunet, S. and Maro, B. (2005) Cytoskeleton and cell cycle control during meiotic maturation of the mouse oocyte: integrating time and space. *Reproduction*, 130, 801–811.

Catt, S.L., Catt, J.W., Gomez, M.C., Maxwell, W.M. and Evans, G. (1996) Birth of a male lamb derived from an in vitro matured oocyte fertilised by intracytoplasmic injection of a single presumptive male sperm. *Vet. Rec*., 139, 494–495.

Chung, J.T., Keefer, C.L. and Downey, B.R. (2000) Activation of bovine oocytes following intracytoplasmic sperm injection (ICSI). *Theriogenology*, 53, 1273–1284.

Cochran, R., Meintjes, M., Reggio, B., Hylan, D., Carter, J., Pinto, C., Paccamonti, D. and Godke, R. (1998) Live foals produced from sperm-injected oocytes derived from pregnant mares. *J. Equine Vet. Sci*., 18, 736–740.

Comizzoli, P., Marquant-Le Guienne, B., Heyman, Y. and Renard, J.P. (2000) Onset of the first S-phase is determined by a paternal effect during the G1-phase in bovine zygotes. *Biol. Reprod.,* 62, 1677–1684.

Cox, G.F., Bürger, J., Lip, V., Mau, U.A., Sperling, K., Wu, B.L. and Horsthemke, B. (2002) Intracytoplasmic sperm injection may increase the risk of imprinting defects. *Am. J. Hum. Genet*., 71, 162–164.

Dean, W., Santos, F., Stojkovic, M., Zakhartchenko, V., Walter, J., Wolf, E. and Reik, W. (2001) Conservation of methylation reprogramming in mammalian development: aberrant reprogramming in cloned embryos. *Proc. Natl. Acad. Sci. USA*, 98, 13734–13738.

De Rosa, A., Attanasio, L., Boccia, L., Pellerano, G., Campanile, G. and Gasparrini, B. (2007) Cryotop vitrification for in vitro-produced buffalo (*Bubalus bubalis*) embryos. *Reprod. Fertil. Dev*., 19, 174–175.

Devito, L.G., Fernandes, C.B., Blanco, I.D.P., Tsuribe, P.M. and Landim-Alvarenga, F.C. (2010) Use of a piezo drill for intracytoplasmic sperm injection into cattle oocytes activated with ionomycin associated with roscovitine. *Reprod. Domest. Anim*., 45, 654–658.

Dinnyés, A., Carolan, C., Lonergan, P., Massip, A. and Mermillod, P. (1996) Survival of frozen or vitrified bovine blastocysts produced in vitro in synthetic oviduct fluid. *Theriogenology*, 46, 1425–1439.

Dinnyés, A., Lonergan, P., Fair, T., Boland, M.P. and Yang, X. (1999) Timing of the first cleavage post-insemination affects cryosurvival of in vitro-produced bovine blastocysts. *Mol. Reprod. Dev.*, 53, 318–324.

Du, Y., Zhang, Y., Li, J., Kragh, P.M., Kuwayama, M., Ieda, S., Zhang, X., Schmidt, M., Bøgh, I.B., Purup, S., Pedersen, A.M., Villemoes, K., Yang, H., Bolund, L. and Vajta, G. (2007) Simplified cryopreservation of porcine cloned blastocysts. *Cryobiology,* 54, 181–187.

Ducibella, T., Huneau, D., Angelichio, E., Xu, Z., Schultz, R.M., Kopf, G.S., Fissore, R., Madoux, S. and Ozil, J.P. (2002) Egg-to-embryo transition is driven by differential responses to Ca^{2+} oscillation number. *Dev. Biol.*, 250, 280–291.

Emuta, C. and Horiuchi, T. (2001) Effects of timing of activation and aging of bovine oocytes fertilized by intracytoplasmic sperm injection (ICSI) on cleavage and subsequent embryonic development in vitro. *J. Reprod. Dev.*, 47, 399–405.

Fissore, R.A., Pinto-Correia, C. and Robl, J.M. (1995) Inositol trisphosphate-induced calcium release in the generation of calcium oscillation in bovine eggs. *Biol. Reprod.*, 53, 766–774.

Fujinami, N., Hosoi, Y., Kato, H., Matsumoto, K., Saeki, K. and Iritani, A. (2004) Activation with ethanol improves embryo development of ICSI-derived oocytes by regulation of kinetics of MPF activity. *J. Reprod. Dev.*, 50, 171–178.

Fulka, H. and Fulka, J. Jr. (2006) No differences in the DNA methylation pattern in mouse zygotes produced in vivo, in vitro, or by intracytoplasmic sperm injection. *Fertil. Steril.,* 86, 1534–1536.

Galli, C., Vassiliev, I., Lagutina, I., Galli, A. and Lazzari, G. (2003) Bovine embryo development following ICSI: effect of activation, sperm capacitation and pre-treatment with dithiothreitol. *Theriogenology*, 60, 1467–1480.

Gautier, J., Minshull, J., Lohka, M., Glotzer, M., Hunt, T. and Maller, J.L. (1990) Cyclin is a component of maturation-promoting factor from Xenopus. *Cell,* 60, 487–494.

George, F., Daniaux, C., Genicot, G., Verhaeghe, B., Lambert, P. and Donnay, I. (2008) Set up of a serum-free culture system for bovine embryos: embryo development and quality before and after transient transfer. *Theriogenology*, 69, 612–623.

Gordo, A.C., Wu, H., He, C.L. and Fissore, R.A. (2000) Injection of sperm cytosolic factor into mouse metaphase II oocytes induces different developmental fates according to the frequency of $[Ca^{2+}]i$ oscillations and oocyte age. *Biol. Reprod.*, 62, 1370–1379.

Goto, K., Kinoshita, A., Takuma, Y. and Ogawa, K. (1990) Fertilisation of bovine oocytes by the injection of immobilised, killed spermatozoa. *Vet. Rec.*, 127, 517–520.

Han, Y.M., Yamashina, H., Koyama, N., Lee, K.K. and Fukui, Y. (1994) Effects of the quality and the developmental stage on the survival of IVF-Derived bovine blastocysts cultured in vitro after freezing and thawing. *Theriogenology*, 42, 645–654.

Hamano, K., Li, X., Qian, X.Q., Funauchi, K., Furudate, M. and Minato, Y. (1999) Gender preselection in cattle with intracytoplasmically injected, flow cytometrically sorted sperm heads. *Biol. Reprod.*, 60, 1194–1197.

Hirabayashi, M., Kato, M., Aoto, T., Sekimoto, A., Ueda, M., Miyoshi, I., Kasai, N. and Hochi S. (2002) Offspring derived from intracytoplasmic injection of transgenic rat sperm. *Transgenic Res.*, 11, 221–228.

Hirabayashi, M., Kato, M., Ishikawa, A., Kaneko, R., Yagi, T. and Hochi, S. (2005) Factors affecting production of transgenic rats by ICSI-mediated DNA transfer: effects of sonication and freeze-thawing of spermatozoa, rat strains for sperm and oocyte donors, and different constructs of exogenous DNA. *Mol. Reprod. Dev.*, 70, 422–428.

Horiuchi, T., Emuta, C., Yamauchi, Y., Oikawa, T., Numabe, T. and Yanagimachi, R. (2002) Birth of normal calves after intracytoplasmic sperm injection of bovine oocytes: a methodological approach. *Theriogenology*, 57, 1013–1024.

Hosoi, Y., Miyake, M., Utsumi, K. and Iritani A. (1988) Development of rabbit oocytes after microinjection of spermatozoa. In: *Proceedings of the 11th International Congress on Animal Reproduction and Artificial Insemination*, 3, 331.

Hoth, M. and Penner, R. (1992) Depletion of intracellular calcium stores activates a calcium current in mast cells. *Nature*, 355, 353–356.

Huo, L.J., Fan, H.Y., Zhong, Z.S., Chen, D.Y., Schatten, H. and Sun, Q.Y. (2004) Ubiquitin-proteasome pathway modulates mouse oocyte meiotic maturation and fertilization via regulation of MAPK cascade and cyclin B1 degradation. *Mech. Dev.*, 121, 1275–1287.

Hwang, S., Lee, E., Yoon, J., Yoon, B.K., Lee, J.H. and Choi, D. (2000) Effects of electric stimulation on bovine oocyte activation and embryo development in intracytoplasmic sperm injection procedure. *J. Assist. Reprod. Genet.*, 17, 310–314.

Jones, K.T. (2005) Mammalian egg activation: from Ca^{2+} spiking to cell cycle progression. *Reproduction,* 130, 813–823.

Katayose, H., Yanagida, K., Shinoki, T., Kawahara, T., Horiuchi, T. and Sato, A. (1999) Efficient injection of bull spermatozoa into oocytes using a piezo-driven pipette. *Theriogenology*, 52, 1215–1224.

Kelly, J.M., Kleemann, D.O., Kuwayama, M. and Walker, S.K. (2004) Vitrification of in vitro-produced bovine and ovine embryos using the minimum volume cooling cryotop method. *Reprod. Fertil. Dev.*, 16, 172–173.

Keskintepe, L. and Brackett, B.G. (2000) Cryopreservation of bovine blastocysts obtained by intracytoplasmic sperm injection. *Theriogenology*, 53, 1041–1052.

Keskintepe, L., Pacholczyk, G., Machnicka, A., Norris, K., Curuk, M.A., Khan, I. and Brackett, B.G. (2002) Bovine blastocyst development from oocytes injected with freeze-dried spermatozoa. *Biol. Reprod.*, 67, 409–415.

Kimura, Y. and Yanagimachi, R. (1995) Intracytoplasmic sperm injection in the mouse. *Biol. Reprod.*, 52, 709–720.

Kuwayama, M. and Kato, O. (2000) All-round vitrification method for human oocytes and embryos. *J. Assist. Reprod. Genet.*, 17, 477.

Laowtammathron, C., Lorthongpanich, C., Ketudat-Cairns, M., Hochi, S. and Parnpai, R. (2005) Factors affecting cryosurvival of nuclear-transferred bovine and swamp buffalo blastocysts: effects of hatching stage, linoleic acid-albumin in IVC medium and Ficoll supplementation to vitrification solution. *Theriogenology*, 64, 1185–1196.

Li, E. (2002) Chromatin modification and epigenetic reprogramming in mammalian development. *Nat. Rev. Genet.*, 3, 662–673.

Li, X, Hamano, K., Qian, X.Q., Funauchi, K., Furudate, M. and Minato, Y. (1999) Oocyte activation and parthenogenetic development of bovine oocytes following intracytoplasmic sperm injection. *Zygote*, 7, 233–237.

Liebermann, J., Nawroth, F., Isachenko, V., Isachenko, E., Rahimi, G. and Tucker, M.J. (2002) Potential importance of vitrification in reproductive medicine. *Biol. Reprod.*, 67, 1671–1680.

Liu, L., Ju, J.C. and Yang, X. (1998) Parthenogenetic development and protein patterns of newly matured bovine oocytes after chemical activation. *Mol. Reprod. Dev.*, 49, 298–307.

Liu, L. and Yang, X. (1999) Interplay of maturation-promoting factor and mitogen-activated protein kinase inactivation during metaphase-to-interphase transition of activated bovine oocytes. *Biol. Reprod.*, 61, 1–7.

Liu, Y., Du, Y., Lin, L., Li, J., Kragh, P.M., Kuwayama, M., Bolund, L., Yang, H. and Vajta, G. (2008) Comparison of the efficiency of open pulled straw (OPS) and Cryotop vitrification for cryopreservation of in vitro matured pig oocytes. *Cryo Letters*, 29, 315–320.

Lu, K.H., Gordon, I., Chen, H.B., Gallagher, M. and McGovern, H. (1988) Birth of twins after transfer of cattle embryos produced by in vitro techniques. *Vet. Rec.*, 122, 539–540.

Lorca, T., Cruzalegui, F.H., Fesquet, D., Cavadore, J.C., Méry, J., Means, A. and Dorée, M. (1993) Calmodulin-dependent protein kinase II mediates inactivation of MPF and CSF upon fertilization of Xenopus eggs. *Nature*, 366, 270–273.

Malcuit, C., Knott, J.G., He, C., Wainwright, T., Parys, J.B., Robl J.M. and Fissore, R.A. (2005) Fertilization and inositol 1,4,5-trisphosphate (IP_3)-induced calcium release in type-1 inositol 1,4,5-trisphosphate receptor down-regulated bovine eggs. *Biol. Reprod.*, 73, 2–13.

Malcuit, C., Kurokawa, M. and Fissore, R.A. (2006a) Calcium oscillations and mammalian egg activation. *J. Cell Physiol.*, 206, 565–573.

Malcuit, C., Maserati, M., Takahashi, Y., Page, R. and Fissore, R.A. (2006b) Intracytoplasmic sperm injection in the bovine induces abnormal $[Ca^{2+}]i$ responses and oocyte activation. *Reprod. Fertil. Dev.*, 18, 39–51.

Martin, M.J. (2000) Development of in vivo-matured porcine oocytes following intracytoplasmic sperm injection. *Biol. Reprod.*, 63, 109–112.

Massip, A., Mermillod, P. and Dinnyes, A. (1995) Morphology and biochemistry of in-vitro produced bovine embryos: implications for their cryopreservation. *Hum. Reprod.*, 10, 3004–3011.

McAvey, B.A., Wortzman, G.B., Williams, C.J. and Evans, J.P. (2002) Involvement of calcium signaling and the actin cytoskeleton in the membrane block to polyspermy in mouse eggs. *Biol. Reprod.*, 67, 1342–1352.

McLay, D.W. and Clarke, H.J. (1997) The ability to organize sperm DNA into functional chromatin is acquired during meiotic maturation in murine oocytes. *Dev. Biol.*, 186, 73–84.

McLay, D.W. and Clarke, H.J. (2003) Remodelling the paternal chromatin at fertilization in mammals. *Reproduction*, 125, 625–633.

Meehan, R.R. (2003) DNA methylation in animal development. *Semin. Cell Dev. Biol.,* 14, 53–65.

Méo, S.C., Leal, C.L. and Garcia, J.M. (2004) Activation and early parthenogenesis of bovine oocytes treated with ethanol and strontium. *Anim. Reprod. Sci*., 81, 35–46.

Morató, R., Izquierdo, D., Paramio, M.T. and Mogas, T. (2008) Cryotops versus open-pulled straws (OPS) as carriers for the cryopreservation of bovine oocytes: effects on spindle and chromosome configuration and embryo development. *Cryobiology*, 57, 137–141.

Morozumi, K., Shikano, T., Miyazaki, S. and Yanagimachi, R. (2006) Simultaneous removal of sperm plasma membrane and acrosome before intracytoplasmic sperm injection improves oocyte activation/embryonic development. *Proc. Natl. Acad. Sci. USA*, 103, 17661–17666.

Morozumi, K. and Yanagimachi, R. (2005) incorporation of the acrosome into the oocytes during intracytoplasmic sperm injection could be potentially hazardous to embryo development. *Proc. Natl. Acad. Sci. USA*, 102, 14209–14214.

Mucci, N., Aller, J., Kaiser, G.G., Hozbor, F., Cabodevila, J. and Alberio, R.H. (2006) Effect of estrous cow serum during bovine embryo culture on blastocyst development and cryotolerance after slow freezing or vitrification. *Theriogenology*, 65, 1551–1562.

Nakada, K., Mizuno, J., Shiraishi, K., Endo, K. and Miyazaki, S. (1995) Initiation, persistence, and cessation of the series of intracellular Ca^{2+} responses during fertilization of bovine eggs. *J. Reprod. Dev*., 41, 77–84.

Nakada, K. and Mizuno, J. (1998) Intracellular calcium responses in bovine oocytes induced by spermatozoa and by reagents. *Theriogenology,* 50, 269–282.

Nakamura, S., Terada, Y., Horiuchi, T., Emuta, C., Murakami, T., Yaegashi, N. and Okamura, K. (2001) Human sperm aster formation and pronuclear decondensation in bovine eggs following intracytoplasmic sperm injection using a Piezo-driven pipette: a novel assay for human sperm centrosomal function. *Biol. Reprod*., 65, 1359–1363.

Navara, C.S., First, N.L. and Schatten, G. (1994) Microtubule organization in the cow during fertilization, polyspermy, parthenogenesis, and nuclear transfer: the role of the sperm aster. *Dev. Biol*., 162, 29–40.

Nedambale, T.L., Dinnyés, A., Groen, W., Dobrinsky, J.R., Tian, X.C. and Yang, X. (2004) Comparison on in vitro fertilized bovine embryos cultured in KSOM or SOF and cryopreserved by slow freezing or vitrification. *Theriogenology*, 62, 437–449.

Neri, Q.V., Takeuchi, T. and Palermo, G.D. (2008) An update of assisted reproductive technologies results in the United States. *Ann. N. Y. Acad. Sci*., 1127, 41–48.

Nikolettos, N., Asimakopoulos, B. and Papastefanou, I.S. (2006) Intracytoplasmic sperm injection -an assisted reproduction technique that should make us cautious about imprinting deregulation. *J. Soc. Gyneco. Investig*., 13, 317–328.

Ock, S.A., Bhak, J.S., Balasubramanian, S., Lee, H.J., Choe, S.Y. and Rho, G.J. (2003) Different activation treatments for successful development of bovine oocytes following intracytoplasmic sperm injection. *Zygote*, 11, 69–76.

Oikawa, T., Takada, N., Kikuchi, T., Numabe, T., Takenaka, M. and Horiuchi, T. (2005) Evaluation of activation treatments for blastocyst production and birth of viable calves following bovine intracytoplasmic sperm injection. *Anim. Reprod. Sci*., 86, 187–194.

Ozil, J.P. and Huneau, D. (2001) Activation of rabbit oocytes: the impact of the Ca^{2+} Signal regime on development. *Development,* 128, 917–928.

Ozil, J.P., Markoulaki, S., Toth, S., Matson, S., Banrezes, B., Knott, J.G., Schultz, R.M., Huneau, D. and Ducibella, T. (2005) Egg activation events are regulated by the duration of a sustained [Ca^{2+}]cyt signal in the mouse. *Dev. Biol.*, 282, 39–54.

Palermo, G., Joris, H., Devroey, P. and Van Steirteghem, A.C. (1992) Pregnancies after intracytoplasmic injection of single spermatozoon into an oocyte. *Lancet*, 340, 17–18.

Park, J.S., Jeong, Y.S., Shin, S.T., Lee, K.K. and Kang, Y.K. (2007) Dynamic DNA methylation reprogramming: active demethylation and immediate remethylation in the male pronucleus of bovine zygotes. *Dev. Dyn.*, 236, 2523–2533.

Park, S.P., Kim, E.Y., Kim, D.I., Park, N.H., Won, Y.S., Yoon, S.H., Chung, K.S. and Lim, J.H. (1999) Simple, efficient and successful vitrification of bovine blastocysts using electron microscope grids. *Hum. Reprod.*, 14, 2838–2843.

Perecin, F., Méo, S.C., Leal, C.L.V. and Garcia, J.M. (2007) Oocyte activation and preimplantation development of bovine embryos obtained by specific inhibition of cyclin-dependent kinases. *Arq. Bras. Med. Vet. Zootec.*, 59, 280–287.

Perreault, S.D., Barbee, R.R., Elstein, K.H., Zucker, R.M. and Keefer, C.L. (1988a) Interspecies differences in the stability of mammalian sperm nuclei assessed in vivo by sperm microinjection and in vitro by flow cytometry. *Biol. Reprod.*, 39, 157–167.

Perreault, S.D., Barbee, R.R. and Slott, V.L. (1988b) Importance of glutathione in the activity and maintenance of sperm nuclear decondensing activity in maturing hamster oocytes. *Dev. Biol.,* 125, 181–186.

Perreault, S.D., Wolff, R.A. and Zirkin, B.R. (1984) The role of disulfide bond reduction during mammalian sperm nuclear decondensation in vivo. *Dev. Biol.*, 101, 160–167.

Perry, A.C., Wakayama, T., Kishikawa, H., Kasai, T., Okabe, M., Toyoda, Y. and Yanagimachi, R. (1999) Mammalian transgenesis by intracytoplasmic sperm injection. *Science,* 284, 1180–1183.

Pope, C.E., Johnson, C.A., McRae, M.A., Keller, G.L. and Dresser, B.L. (1998) Development of embryos produced by intracytoplasmic sperm injection of cat oocytes. *Anim. Reprod. Sci.*, 53, 221–236.

Reik, W., Dean, W. and Walter, J. (2001) Epigenetic reprogramming in mammalian development. *Science*, 293, 1089–1093.

Rho, G.J., Kawarsky, S., Johnson, W.H., Kochhar, K. and Betteridge, K.J. (1998a) Sperm and oocyte treatments to improve the formation of male and female pronuclei and subsequent development following intracytoplasmic sperm injection into bovine oocytes. *Biol. Reprod.*, 59, 918–924.

Rho, G.J., Lee, S.L., Kim, Y.S., Yeo, H.J., Ock, S.A., Balasubramanian, S. and Choe, S.Y. (2004) Intracytoplasmic sperm injection of frozen-thawed bovine oocytes and subsequent embryo development. *Mol. Reprod. Dev.*, 68, 449–455.

Rho, G.J., Wu, B., Kawarsky, S., Leibo, S.P. and Betteridge, K.J. (1998b) Activation regimens to prepare bovine oocytes for intracytoplasmic sperm injection. *Mol. Reprod. Dev.,* 50, 485–492.

Ross, P.J., Beyhan, Z., Lager, A.E., Yoon, S.Y., Malcuit, C., Schellander, K., Fissore, R.A. and Cibelli, J.B. (2008) Parthenogenetic activation of bovine oocytes using bovine and murine phospholipase C zeta. *BMC Dev. Biol.*, 8, 16.

Rougier, N., Bourc'his, D., Gomes, D.M., Niveleau, A., Plachot, M., Pàldi, A. and Viegas-Péquignot, E. (1998) Chromosome methylation patterns during mammalian preimplantation development. *Genes Dev.*, 12, 2108–2113.

Rybouchkin, A., Dozortsev, D., de Sutter, P., Qian, C. and Dhont, M. (1995) Intracytoplasmic injection of human spermatozoa into mouse oocytes: a useful model to investigate the oocyte-activation capacity and the karyotype of human spermatozoa. *Hum. Reprod.*, 10, 1130–1135.

Saha, S., Rajamahendran, R., Boediono, A., Sumantri, C. and Suzuki, T. (1996) Viability of bovine blastocysts obtained after 7, 8 or 9 days of culture in vitro following vitrification and one-step rehydration. *Theriogenology*, 46, 331–343.

Santos, F., Hendrich, B., Reik, W. and Dean, W. (2002) Dynamic reprogramming of DNA methylation in the early mouse embryo. *Dev. Biol.*, 241, 172–182.

Schultz, R.M. and Kopf, G.S. (1995) Molecular basis of mammalian egg activation. *Curr. Top. Dev. Biol.*, 30, 21–62.

Shiina, Y., Kaneda, M., Matsuyama, K., Tanaka, K., Hiroi, M. and Doi, K. (1993) Role of the extracellular Ca^{2+} on the intracellular Ca^{2+} changes in fertilized and activated mouse oocytes. *J. Reprod. Fertil.*, 97, 143–150.

Shin, M.R. and Kim, N.H. (2003) Maternal gamma (γ)-tubulin is involved in microtubule reorganization during bovine fertilization and parthenogenesis. *Mol. Reprod. Dev.*, 64, 438–445.

Shirazi, A., Nazari, H., Ahmadi, E., Heidari, B. and Shams-Esfandabadi, N. (2009) Effect of culture system on survival rate of vitrified bovine embryos produced in vitro. *Cryobiology*, 59, 285–290.

Soloy, E., Kanka, J., Viuff, D., Smith, S.D., Callesen, H. and Greve, T. (1997) Time course of pronuclear deoxyribonucleic acid synthesis in parthenogenetically activated bovine oocytes. *Biol. Reprod.*, 57, 27–35.

Sutovsky, P. and Schatten, G. (1997) Depletion of glutathione during bovine oocyte maturation reversibly blocks the decondensation of the male pronucleus and the pronuclear apposition during fertilization. *Biol. Reprod.*, 56, 1503–1512.

Tatham, B.G., Sathananthan, A.H., Dharmawardena, V., Munesinghe, D.Y., Lewis, I. and Trounson, A.O. (1996) Centrifugation of bovine oocytes for nuclear micromanipulation and sperm microinjection. *Hum. Reprod.*, 11, 1499–1503.

Telford, N.A., Watson, A.J. and Schultz, G.A. (1990) Transition from maternal to embryonic control in early mammalian development: a comparison of several species. *Mol. Reprod. Dev.*, 26, 90–100.

Uehara, T. and Yanagimachi, R. (1976) Microsurgical injection of spermatozoa into hamster eggs with subsequent transformation of sperm nuclei into male pronuclei. *Biol. Reprod.*, 15, 467–470.

Ushijima, H. and Nakane, T. (2006) Present status and prospects for bovine intracytoplasmic sperm injection with in vitro-matured oocytes and frozen semen. *J. Mammal. Ova Res.*, 23, 107–113.

Van Soom, A., Ysebaert, M.T. and de Kruif, A. (1997) Relationship between timing of development, morula morphology, and cell allocation to inner cell mass and trophectoderm in in vitro-produced bovine embryos. *Mol. Reprod. Dev.*, 47, 47–56.

Vajta, G. and Kuwayama, M. (2006) Improving cryopreservation systems. *Theriogenology,* 65, 236–244.

Vajta, G., Rindom, N., Peura, T.T., Holm, P., Greve, T. and Callesen, H. (1999) The effect of media, serum and temperature on in vitro survival of bovine blastocysts after Open Pulled Straw (OPS) vitrification. *Theriogenology,* 52, 939–948.

Vernaeve, V., Bonduelle, M., Tournaye, H., Camus, M., Van Steirteghem, A. and Devroey, P. (2003) Pregnancy outcome and neonatal data of children born after ICSI using testicular sperm in obstructive and non-obstructive azospermia. *Hum. Reprod.*, 18, 2093–2097.

Vincent, C., Pickering, S.J. and Johnson, M.H. (1990) The hardening effect of dimethylsulphoxide on the mouse zona pellucida requires the presence of an oocyte and is associated with a reduction in the number of cortical granules present. *J. Reprod. Fertil.,* 89, 253–259.

Wall, R.J. and Hawk, H.W. (1988) Development of centrifuged cow zygotes cultured in rabbit oviduct. *J. Reprod Fertil.,* 82, 673–680.

Wei, H. and Fukui, Y. (2000) Technical improvement in intracytoplasmic sperm injection (ICSI) in cattle. *J. Reprod. Dev.*, 46, 403–407.

Wei, H. and Fukui, Y. (2002) Births of calves derived from embryos produced by intracytoplasmic sperm injection without exogenous oocyte activation. *Zygote,* 10, 149–153.

Westhusin, M.E., Anderson, J.G., Harms, P.G. and Kraemer, D.C. (1984) Microinjection of spermatozoa into bovine eggs. *Theriogenology,* 21, 274.

Wilkins, J.F. (2005) Genomic imprinting and methylation: epigenetic canalization and conflict. *Trends Genet.*, 21, 356–365.

Winger, Q.A., De La Fuente, R., King, W.A., Armstrong, D.T. and Watson, A.J. (1997) Bovine parthenogenesis is characterized by abnormal chromosomal complements: implications for maternal and paternal co-dependence during early bovine development. *Dev. Genet.*, 21, 160–166.

Wu, C.-t. and Morris, J.R. (2001) Gene, genetics and epigenetics: a correspondence. *Science,* 293, 1103–1105.

Wu, H., He, C.L. and Fissore, R.A. (1997) Injection of a porcine sperm factor triggers calcium oscillations in mouse oocytes and bovine eggs. *Mol. Reprod. Dev.*, 46, 176–189.

Wu, H., Smyth, J., Luzzi, V., Fukami, K., Takenawa, T., Black, S.L., Allbritton, N.L. and Fissore, R.A. (2001) Sperm factor induce intracellular free calcium oscillations by stimulating the phosphoinositide pathway. *Biol. Reprod.*, 64, 1338–1349.

Yamauchi, Y., Yanagimachi, R. and Horiuchi, T. (2002) Full-term development of golden hamster oocytes following intracytoplasmic sperm head injection. *Biol. Reprod.*, 67, 534–539.

Yoshida, N. and Perry, A.C.F. (2007) Piezo-actuated mouse intracytoplasmic sperm injection (ICSI). *Nat. Protoc.*, 2, 296–304.

In: In Vitro Fertilization
Editor: Samantha P. Steiger, pp. 65-81

ISBN 978-1-61209-961-3

Chapter III

Paediatric Outcomes of Artificial Reproductive Technologies: Lessons from Research

John R. Apps and Alastair G. Sutcliffe
Institute of Child Health, UCL, General Paediatric and Adolescent Unit, London, WC1N 1EH, UK

Abstract

Over 3,500,000 people have been born using Assisted Reproductive Technologies (ART).

This chapter reviews the existing research into the health of this population, highlights uncertainties and attempts to draw lessons for future practice and research.

The introduction of artificial methods to augment an already complex biological phenomenon increases the potential for adverse outcomes.

Much of the adverse outcome relates to morbidity of higher order pregnancies. Early studies were methodologically limited, however as larger, better designed studies and meta-analyses are published it has become clear that ART children have higher rates of preterm birth, low birth weight and slightly higher rates of congenital anomalies.

As existing cohorts get older, evidence regarding longer term biological and sociological outcomes is increasing. Whilst generally reassuring, showing little or no difference in

growth, physical health, neurological, neuro-developmental, and psychosocial wellbeing, further research and longer follow up into both adolescent and adult life is required for these and other outcomes.

As newer techniques are developed and become more widespread it will be important to establish prospective surveillance to identify and reduce adverse outcome risk.

Introduction

Over 3,500,000 people have been born as a result of Artificial Reproductive Technologies (ART), with about 1-3% of children born in developed countries being conceived in this way [1,2]. Early research focussed predominantly on Obstetric outcomes and so it is only recently that Paediatric outcomes are becoming understood.

Paediatric outcomes have implications both for informing potential parents adequately prior to undergoing ART and considering the health economics of caring for high dependency neonates and children.

Increasingly, epidemiological and basic science data demonstrate effects changes in the early environment of the unborn child can have on long term health [3,4]. Deciphering such risk from confounding factors is methodologically challenging. Parents undergoing IVF are on average older, more highly educated and less likely to smoke than the general parent population [5]. In addition, the impact of infertility itself on outcome is increasingly recognised as contributing to some adverse outcomes, though is as yet poorly understood [1,2].

This chapter reviews the current evidence regarding peri-natal and longer term paediatric outcomes and attempts to draw lessons for both future practice and research.

Multiple Pregnancy

ART has been associated with a surge in multiple pregnancies, and with it adverse outcomes. It is associated with an approximately 20 fold increased risk of twins and 400 fold increased risk of higher order pregnancies [6]. ART has multiple birth rates between 22.7% and 31% in the UK and the USA and contributes 21% of all multiple births in the UK, compared to only 1.2% of singletons. [1,7]

Multiple births are associated with an increased risk of preterm birth, low birth weight (50% <2500g compared to 6% in singletons), neonatal mortality (46.8/1000 compared to 8.8% for IVF singletons) congenital malformation and disability among survivors (1 in 13 twins, 1 in 5 triplets) as well as a considerable health economic expenditure [8,9,10].

Single Embryo Transfer

There is now good evidence from clinical trials and a recent Cochrane review that an approach using an initial transfer of a single embryo, followed if necessary by transfer of a cryopreserved embryo, a technique known as Single Embryo Transfer (SET), results in a similar live birth rate (OR 0.81 (95%CI 0.59-1.11)) compared to dual embryo transfer (DET) whilst significantly lowering the multiple birth rate (OR=0.04 (95% CI 0.01-0.11))[10].

Neonatal outcomes are also improved, with a Scandinavian randomised control trial finding that SET was associated with significantly less preterm births, low birth weight neonates, and lower neonatal hospitalisation compared to DET with considerable health economic savings. [11]. SET has now become the mandated norm in some countries, such as Sweden, where multiple birth rates are around 5%, with pregnancy rates maintained at 30-

40%, per transfer [2]. Wider usage of this technique has the potential to greatly reduce the morbidity associated with ART multiple pregnancies.

Perinatal Outcome

Singletons

Several large meta-analyses have shown an increased risk of pre-term birth, low birth weight, small for gestational age and perinatal mortality among ART singletons when controlled for parental age and parity (Table I) [12,13,14]. More recent population based studies echo these including a large American study using their register of ART births [15].

Table I.

	Adverse outcomes: ART singletons compared to spontaneously conceived controls (adapted from 1)					
Study:	No ART Conceived infants	Preterm birth (PTB) (<37weeks)	Low Birth Weight (LBW) (<2500g)	Very low birth weight (VLBW) (1500g)	Small for gestational age (SGA) or Intrauterine Growth Restriction (IUGR)	Perinatal mortality
Jackson et al, 2004 Meta-analysis [12]	12,283	OR 2.0 (95%CI 1.7-2.2)	OR 1.8 (95% CI 1.4-2.2)	OR 2.7 (95% CI 2.3-3.1)	SGA: OR 1.6 (95% CI 1.3-2.0)	OR2.2 (95%CI 1.6-3.0)
Helmerhorst et al, 2004, Meta-analysis [13]	5361	RR 3.0 (95%CI 2.1-4.3)	RR 1.4 (95%CI 1.2-1.7)	RR 3.0 (95% CI 2.1-4.4)	SGA: RR 1.5 (95% CI 1.4-1.7)	RR 1.7 (95% CI 1.1-2.5)
McDonald et al 2010, Meta-analysis [14]	31 032	RR 1.84 (95% CI 1.54-2.21)	RR 1.60 (95%CI 1.29-1.98)	RR 2.65 (95%CI 1.83-3.84)	IUGR: RR 1.45 95% CI 1.04-2.00	Not available
Schieve et al, 2004, Large US register based study	62 551	RR 1.4 (95% CI 1.3-1.5)	RR 1.6 (95% CI 1.5-1.8)	RR 1.8 (95% CI 1.5-1.9)	Not available	Not available

Understanding the aetiology of this adverse outcome is a challenge.

Term ART babies are also of a lower birth weight, consequently differences in obstetric monitoring and a suggested earlier threshold for delivery intervention among ART pregnancies cannot explain this [15].

Early fetal loss in a twin pregnancy, resulting in a singleton, occurs in 8.8% of ART singleton pregnancies and it has been suggested this may contribute to the increased adverse outcomes [15]. Luke et al studied over 22,000 ART singleton births and identified 1727 where 2 or 3 foetal heart beats had been identified in the first trimester. These pregnancies were significantly more likely to be preterm and have low birth weight compared to those ART pregnancies which did not suffer early fetal loss [16]. However, Schieve et al's US register based study found increased LBW, VLBW, Preterm delivery, preterm LBW and term

LBW remained despite limiting analysis to pregnancies with only one heart beat in the first trimester [15].

The role of infertility in contributing to adverse outcome is also debated. There is evidence that children of parents who have taken over 12 months to conceive spontaneously are at increased risk of adverse outcome [17,18] as are those born by non IVF techniques such as Ovarian Stimuation or Artificial Insemination [19]. Several studies have compared ART children with such 'infertile' controls. De Geyter et al, 2006, compared outcomes of IVF and ICSI births with infertile couples (time to pregnancy greater than 1yr) who conceived without the need for IVF/ICSI/IUI or cryopreservation and found that birth weight and gestational duration was significantly less in infants conceived by ICSI or IVF [20]. However, when compared with sibling matched controls statistical significance was lost for IVF children, though numbers were small and the power limited (20%) [20]. Such a loss of significance when comparing ART children with spontaneously conceived siblings was also found in a registry based study of singletons [21]. Whilst overall comparison between groups (n= 2204 in each group) found that there was statistically lower mean birth weight, shorter gestation, a higher risk of small for gestational age and increased perinatal mortality among ART children such differences were lost when paired analysis between siblings was performed; perinatal mortality was actually decreased in ART siblings OR 0.36 (0.20-0.67) [21]. This study has been criticised as it is possible that some sibling controls were born using ART techniques.[21]

A Swedish study comparing outcomes across 25 years from 1982-2006 has found a decreasing rate of adverse preterm birth and low birth weight when limited to studying singletons, whilst the aetiology of this is unclear it has been suggested this may relate to changes in the characteristics of mothers undergoing IVF. [5]

Collectively these studies highlight the importance of parental factors (especially the underlying sub-fertility) in determining peri-natal outcome and also the need for careful selection of controls and interpretation of results.

Twins

Several Meta-analyses have compared the peri-natal outcomes of ART twins against spontaneously conceived controls [13, 22, 23]. The most recent of these, McDonald et al, 2010, found an increased risk of preterm birth (RR1.23 (95% CI 1.09-1.41)), low birth weight (1.14 (95% CI 0.06-1.22) as well as shorter mean duration of gestation and mean birth weight among ART twins [22]. Earlier studies and meta-analyses found conflicting and inconsistent results. [13, 23].

Only 1-2% of ART twins are mono-chorionic compared to 22% of naturally conceived twins [24]. Such twins have a higher risk of adverse outcome than di-zygotic twin, however only a few studies have attempted to control for this discrepancy. A large Danish study found an increased risk of prematurity, low birth weight and admission to an intensive care unit in ART twins of unlike sex compared to controls. Whilst differences in rates of prematurity and low birth weight disappeared when controlled for maternal age and parity admission to a neonatal intensive care unit remained significantly more common in ART twins [24]. A recent Australian study found that when comparing all ART twins to spontaneously conceived twins of unlike sex, ART twins were at increased risk of premature delivery, low birth weight, perinatal death and duration of admission after birth [25]. The differences persisted, but were less, when compared to all naturally conceived twins. However this study was limited by several confounding factors. A large Swedish registry study has also recently found increased premature delivery amongst IVF dizygotic twins, though differences in birth weight were lost when controlled for maternal age and parity [26]. These studies again highlight the importance of appropriate and careful selection of controls populations and the challenges in interpreting effects of ART.

Cryopreservation

An increasing proportion of ART births follow freezing of the embryo, approximately 25% worldwide, and up to 40% in some countries [27]. A recent systematic review has compared outcomes of such children with those born following fresh embryo transfer. The majority of studies included found no increase in prematurity, low birth weight or perinatal morbidity, in fact several showed improved outcomes in those undergoing cryopreservation [27].

Congenital Anomalies/Malformations

A possible link between ART and congenital anomalies was raised in 1987 when Lancaster et al reported increased Spina Bifida and Transposition of the Great Arteries following ART [28]. Since then a large number of studies have been performed with conflicting results. Differences in definitions, a lack of consistency in age of examination, the inclusion of stillborns, heterogenous cohorts and lack of appropriate controls and potential confounding limit many of these studies.

It has, however, become increasingly clear that ART is associated with an increased rate of at least some congenital anomalies.

Hansen et al's, 2005 meta-analysis identified seven studies, most of which were large blinded population based studies with clear definitions of birth defect, and found an increased odds ratio for congenital anomalies of 1.40 (95% CI 1.28-1.53) (29). Similarly a 2004 meta-analysis of 19 studies showed a pooled odd's ratio of 1.29 (95% CI 1.01-1.67), though subgroup analyses separating for singleton vs multiple or IVF vs ICSI gave non-significant results [30]. Subsequently a large register based study in the USA has also shown an increased risk among ART singletons for several anomalies, but no increased risk among ART multiple births [31].

The majority of studies group congenital anomalies into heterogenous categories making it hard to interpret exactly which anomalies are at increased risk. Whilst individual studies have differed in their results, certain patterns have emerged with congenital heart disease [31,32,33,34,35], musculoskeletal [32,33] and chromosomal [32, 33] anomalies repeatedly at increased risk. Several studies have also shown an increased risk of urogenital abnormalities in boys, particularly hypospadias. [32, 33, 36, 37, 38], Early studies had suggested this was particularly among ICSI infants compared to standard IVF, however others failed to reproduce this and many of the studies were methodologically limited [32,37,38]. Two meta-analyses have compared birth defects in children conceived by ICSI with standard IVF and found no significant increase in anomalies including urogenital anomalies [39,40].

Multiple pregnancy is a risk factor for congenital anomalies. However the impact of ART is less clear than for singletons, with several studies showing no increase risk of anomalies as a result of ART, including when controlling for zygosity. [29, 30, 31,41]. One study, Klemetti et al, found an overall decreased risk among multiple ART girls (OR 0.5 (95%CI 0.2-0.9)) compared to naturally conceived twins [36].

The majority of studies comparing cryopreserved vs fresh embryos have found no difference in congenital malformation rates [27].

As with birth weight and prematurity, understanding the aetiology of this increased risk is a challenge. Zhu et al compared malformation rates between spontaneously conceived infants who were conceived within or after twelve months of attempting pregnancy with those resulting from ART [41]. An increased risk of malformations was found in singletons spontaneously conceived after greater than 12 months and those undergoing ART (>12mths vs <12mths OR 1.20 (95%CI 1.07-1.35), ART vs <12mths OR1.35 (95%CI 1.23-1.57), however there was no significant difference when ART children were compared to those who had been conceived after twelve months (OR 1.17 (95% CI 1.00-1.35)). Subgroup analysis did show a significant increase in urogenital anomalies in the ART group compared to those taking greater than 12 months to naturally conceive (OR 2.32 (95%CI 1.24-4.35). There was no difference in twins.

Imprinting Disorders

Imprinting refers to when the phenotype of an allele is dependent on which parent it was inherited from, as a result of epigenetic modification. Pre-implantation embryos undergo significant epigenetic remodelling and it has been shown that difference can occur as a result of in vitro manipulation [3]. A number of human conditions, including Beckwith Wiederman syndrome (BWS), Angelman Syndrome (AS) and Prader-Willi syndrome (PWS) can result from abnormal expression of imprinted genes, either through uniparental disomy, deletion, or through epigenetic changes such as alterations in methylation status. Several registry based studies have found an increased risk of Beckwith Wiederman syndrome with ART [42]. The most recent of these, Sutcliffe et al, 2006, contacted families known to regional genetic services or disease support groups to assess the prevalence of ART among such populations [43]. This study found a statistically increased frequency of ART in children with BWS (2.9% (95% CI 1.4-6.3) vs 0.8% expected) though not for PWS. All the ART cases of BWS had lost maternal methylation of the KvDMR1 gene, compared to an expected 50% . Similarly five of seven cases of AS conceived by ICSI had abnormal methylation, whereas AS is usually related to abnormal copy number. Such mechanistic associations further indicate the potential for an increased risk of imprinting disorders with ART.

In contrast a population based study [44] of all children born in Denmark between 1995 and 2002 found no cases of imprinting disorders among the ART population in national disease registers. In this study misclassification may have lead to cases being missed, as indicated by the low prevalence of imprinting disorders in the general population in this study.

The relationship between ART, imprinting and cancer is further discussed in another chapter.

Longer Term Outcomes

Though as yet less studied than perinatal outcomes, there is an increasing literature regarding the outcomes of ART children into childhood. Different study designs, inclusion criteria, and outcome measurements make comparison of studies difficult and limit the opportunity for meta-analyses. Similarly deciphering the aetiology of adverse outcomes is challenging, with the need for controlling for different adverse peri-natal outcomes, ART techniques and fertility problems. Despite ART having been available for over 30 years no studies have as yet extended into adulthood and the impact of ART of future fertility remains largely unknown.

Physical Growth

Studies of height, weight, head circumference and physical examination among IVF and/or ICSI children up to 18mths [45], 3yrs [46], 5yrs [37], 8yrs [47,48], 12yrs [49] and 13 yrs [50] have found no differences, and led Ludwig et al, in a systematic review in 2006 to conclude that there is sufficient evidence that ART children have no difference in physical development [51].

In contrast Koivurova et al, 2003, studying found IVF children to be significantly lighter up to 3 yrs of age and Miles et al, 2007 in a small study in New Zealand found that, when controlled for mid parental height, pre-pubertal children were significantly taller than controls with higher levels of serum IFG2, IGF and IGF binding protein, as well as higher HDL cholesterol and lower triglycerides [52, 53].

A Dutch study of anthropomorphic measurements in older children, between 8 and 16 years found that whilst there was no difference in height, weight, or pubertal stages, fat distribution was significantly different in IVF children [54]. IVF children had more peripheral skinfolds ($p=0.014$), and a lower subscapular-triceps skinfold ratio ($p=0.010$) compared to controls, though other measurements, (sum of truncal skinfolds, total skinfolds, BMI) were not significantly different. Studying the same cohort, Ceelan et al, 2008, found that IVF children had statistically significantly higher systolic and diastolic blood pressures ($p<0.001$),were more likely to be in the top quartile for blood pressure and have a higher fasting blood glucose ($p<0.005$) than spontaneously conceived controls [55]. These differences could not be explained by body size, birth weight, perinatal, parental or subfertility factors. The Dutch famine study has highlighted the importance of early development in affecting cardiovascular disease risk and these findings suggest that ART techniques could also affect this [56]. Further studies, particularly into adulthood are required to further define any such risk.

Studies of hearing and visual impairment have been reassuring showing no significant difference [51]

Health

Studies investigating childhood illnesses and health care utilisation among the ART population have yielded inconsistent findings, likely reflecting variations in study designs, study populations, sizes and outcome measures. The general message emerging from these studies is reassuring. Neurological and neurodevelopmental outcomes will be examined separately in later sections and the relationship between ART and childhood cancer is examined in a separate chapter.

The vast majority of studies have found no difference incidences of childhood illness [57, 47, 48, 45, 60, 58, 59] or hospital admission [45,47,48,61]. However others, including two large population based studies have found increased illness and healthcare utilisation among ART children. [57, 62, 63, 37]

A large registry based study, Kallen et al, found increased hospital admissions among ART children up to six years of age, even when limited to term singletons (OR 1.13 (95%CI 1.06-1.20)) [62]. Discharge diagnoses of behavioural problems, upper respiratory tract infections, asthma/bronchitis and any accident were higher in ART children than controls, despite for adjusting for year of birth, maternal age, parity, smoking and years of unwanted childlessness. Similarly a Finnish cohort study found increased hospital usage among IVF singletons up to 3 years, particularly with respiratory diseases and diarrhoea [52]. Follow up at 7 years found these IVF children were significantly more likely to be admitted to hospital (mean 1.76 vs 1.07 $p<0.0001$) and spend longer in hospital (mean 4.31 days vs 2.61 $p<0.0001$) than controls (64). Post neonatal hospital care cost estimations were 2.6 times greater for IVF singletons and 0.7 times greater for ART twins compared to spontaneously conceived controls. A more recent Finnish cohort study has also found increased admission and duration of hospital stay among ART children [65].

Bonduelle et al, 2005, using a structured interview found that ART children were more likely to have suffered from a significant childhood illness by the age of 5 years, require admission to hospital and received therapy (such as physiotherapy or speech and language therapy) [37]. This study included singletons born at greater than 32 weeks gestation but did not control for differences in peri-natal outcomes between populations. This study also found an increased rate of surgery (24% ICSI, 22%IVF, 14% controls $p=0.001$), particularly minor ear surgery and urogenital surgery among ART children (ICSI 5%, 3% IVF, 1% controls $p<0.005$). Similarly a German cohort study has similarly found an increased incidence of urogenital surgery among ICSI children (19.2% vs 8.9% controls $p=0.013$) particularly for an undescended testicle ($p=0.031$) [57]. Such findings, correlating long term outcomes with findings from studies of peri-natal outcomes, such as congenital anomalies aids in understanding and appreciating adverse outcomes.

Neurological Outcome

A meta-analysis of studies of Cerebral Palsy (CP) in ART children found an overall increased risk of CP (OR 2.18 (95%CI 1.71-2.77) [66]. Limiting analysis to singletons the increased risk was maintained, but not when limited to twins. Of the studies included two large Finnish and Danish cohorts [65,67], both found when controlled for preterm birth the increased risk of CP was lost. In one 88% of cases of CP were born prematurely [65]. A more recent study of Danish births has echoed these findings with differences lost when controlled for gestation and birth weight. [68]. In contrast Lidegaard et al, also studying Danish births, but using different sources for diagnosis and a different analytical approach, found the increased risk of cerebral palsy was maintained when controlling for preterm birth [44].

Two overlapping Swedish population studies have found increased admissions for epilepsy ((OR: 1.5, (95% CI 1.10-2.15))(OR: 1.52, (95%CI 1.30-1.92)) though one lost statistical significance if limited to term children, or adjused for various maternal factors (years of unwanted childlessness, parity, age, smoking) [62,63]. Sun et al found that children born as a result of IVF and ICSI had an increased risk of presentation to hospital with epilepsy (OR 1.83 1.09-3.06) (69). In addition they found children born spontaneously to sub-fertile couples (time to conception >12moths) also had an increased risk (OR 1.38 (95% CI 1.00-1.89)) compared to fertile couples (conceiving within 6months). Statistical difference for both these groups was lost when controlled for preterm birth.

Understanding overall risks are important for counselling potential parents prior to ART, however these studies highlight the importance of controlling for multiple births, neonatal outcomes and parental and infertility factors, when investigating the contribution of the ART towards adverse long term outcomes.

The rarity of cerebral palsy and epilepsy necessarily require studies of thousands of children to clarify any increased risks of ART. Whilst several prospective cohorts have also investigated neurological outcome in ART children aged 5-8 the largest compared only 540ICSI, 437 IVF and 548 naturally conceived children and so lacked statistical precision [37,47,48,57]. Careful design of such studies, and prospective power calculations are therefore crucial in avoiding type 2 errors.

Neurodevelopment

Many studies have investigated the neuro-developmental outcome of ART children with again the vast majority being reassuring. Differences in size, inclusion criteria, age at assessment and assessment tools make it once again difficult to compare these studies.

One population study, Stromberg et al, has investigated developmental delay identified from rehabilitation clinics and found that whilst as a whole ART children aged 1.5 to 14 years had a fourfold increased risk of developmental delay (OR 4.0 (95% CI1.9-8.3)) this difference was lost when analysis was restricted to comparing singletons or twins [70]. This study identified risk factors for suspected developmental delay as low birth weight and low gestational age. This highlights the potential benefit of single embryo transfer techniques in limiting adverse outcomes later in life.

Considering cohort studies with greater than 100 in each group, Sutcliffe et al using Griffiths Mental Development Scales found no difference in between 208 ICSI singletons and 221 spontaneously conceived controls at 1-2 yrs [71] Similarly Koivorova et al did not find any difference in psychomotor development, as assessed using modified Bayley scales between 299 IVF and 558 controls at 12months, 18mths, 2yrs and 3yrs [72]. Ponjaert-Kristoffsen et al in a study across five European countries and comparing singetons born at greater than 32weeks gestation found no difference in Welscher scales of intelligence and McCarthy motor scales between 511ICSI, 424 IVF and 488 spontaneously conceived controls at 5yrs age and Ludwig et al found similar results at 5.5yrs using Zimmer / Volkamer test of motor function and the Kaufman-Assessment Battery to test intelligence [73, 57].

Of studies showing concern, Bowen et al found lower Bayley's score at 1yr among ART children, however this study has been heavily criticized and follow up at 5yr found no difference [74, 61, 51]. Knoester et al's study of 86ICSI, 83IVF and 85 spontaneously conceived 5 year old singletons found statistically lower mean IQ in ICSI children than controls, though not for IVF [75]. This study is limited in size, the use of multiple examiners and lack of control for parental education. When controlled for parental education other similar studies have lost significance [59].

Two studies have investigated the development of children who underwent primplantation genetic diagnosis/screening (PGD), Banerjee et al found no diffence in Griffiths Mental Development Scoring between 49 PGD children and 66 controls aged 3 months to 4 years and Nekkerbroek et al found similar mental and psychomotor outcomes between 70 PGD, 70ICSI and 70 spontaneously conceived controls [76,77].

Overall, these studies have led a systematic review to conclude that there is sufficient evidence to support there is no difference in development of ART children compared to spontaneously conceived children [66].

A number of studies have also investigated autistic spectrum disorders in relation to ART, a systematic review found inconsistent findings across ten studies, the majority showing no difference, one showing an increase among ART children and another a protective effect [66).

Psychosocial Development and Family Dynamics

The artificial and intrusive nature of artificial reproductive technologies and the associated stress has led to theoretical concerns regarding the psychosocial outcome and family dynamics of ART families.

Of the population studies described above only one, Kallen et al, found increased admissions for behavioural problems (OR1.74 (95% CI 1.11-2.74)) among ART children up to 6 years [62]. Whilst Klemetti et al found an overall increased risk of behavioural disorders up to 2 years of age (OR 1.68 (95% CI 1.11-2.53) statistical significance was lost when separated into singleton or twins (Singleton OR1.05 (95% CI 0.57–1.91) Twins OR 3.05 (95%CI 0.70–13.29)) [65]. Other population studies have found no differences [44,70].

A number of smaller cohort studies have been designed to specifically investigate these outcomes using a range of questionnaire and interview based outcome measures. Golombok et al studied a cohort of 102 IVF families, 94 donor insemination families, 102 adoptive families and 102 spontaneously conceived families initially for 4-8 years and then in a follow up study until 12 years and found no difference in incidence of psychiatric disorders or behavioural problems, and that mothers of IVF children reported less stress than spontaneously conceived controls and expressed greater warmth towards their child [78, 79]. Another, larger European study has found similar results comparing 436 IVF, 540 ICSI children and 542 spontaneously conceived controls with no difference regarding parental mental health problems, stress, marital discord or emotional and behavioural problems in children being found (80). No difference was found between feelings of ART and SC children towards their mothers but ISCI mothers reported fewer negative, rejecting or aggressive feelings towards their children and ICSI children expressed more positive feelings towards fathers than controls. Another study of ICSI children also found positive results with fewer behavioural problems and reduced stress in parents when 300 ICSI children aged 5 years were compared to spontaneously conceived controls [81]. In contrast, whilst a small Dutch study found no difference in parental reported behavioural problems between 87 ICSI children, 92 IVF and 85 SC children they found ICSI parents experienced more stress than controls, though this may have resulted from selection bias [82]. One small study of PGD children has also been reassuring with no difference regarding parental stress and PGD parents exhibiting more warmth, and less aggression and rejection towards their children than SC controls [76].

These studies show a reassuring picture, however as yet none have studied outcomes into the more tempestuous area of adolescent family dynamics.

Lessons from Research

Across all these studies a number of key lessons have emerged, both with respect to the outcomes of ART children but also towards the approaches used to investigate them.

Multiple pregnancy is the largest factor contributing towards adverse outcomes seen throughout all categories examined in this review. There now exists a safe, cost effective approach called Single Embryo Transfer to limit this. Wider usage of SET will hopefully reduce adverse outcomes in the future.

As a result of the impact of multiple births, it is important that studies effectively controls for difference in multiple birth rates between ART and control populations, as seen in many of the studies which lost significance when analyses were limited to singleton or multiples. Similarly, when investigating multiple births careful selection of controls to match for chorionicity is needed to avoid erroneous conclusions.

From large studies and meta-analyses it has become clear that singletons, and to a lesser extent multiple birth ART children have an increased rate of adverse perinatal outcome compared to the population. Similarly there is good evidence of an increased risk of congenital anomalies, particularly urogenital anomalies in boys. Understanding the aetiology of this remains a significant challenge, in particular the impact of underlying infertility.

Correlation of congenital anomalies with longer term outcomes such as requirement for surgery will help define risks. Molecular techniques can also aid in determining the contribution of ART to adverse outcomes, as seen in Sutcliffe et al's molecular characterisation of imprinting disorders [43]. There currently appears to be little difference between ART techniques.

For many outcomes, including congenital anomalies, the variations in study designs, outcome measures, inclusion and exclusion criteria and analytical approaches makes it difficult to directly compare apparently conflicting conclusions. Outcome data has been used from a variety of sources, but in many cases the registries/database used were formed for other uses and data quality can be limited and key information regarding confounding factors missing. In addition, for many outcomes, such as for imprinting disorders and specific anomalies, their rarity necessarily requires a large population or registry based approach to detect any increased risk. The application of small underpowered cohort studies raises the potential for type 1 and 2 errors and so these should be interpreted with extreme caution. This rarity also generates the paradox that any increased risk can only be detected once a large number of children have been born. With the development of newer and more invasive techniques, well designed prospective strategies of data collection and analysis will need to be employed to recognise any increased risk and require good collaboration between Obstetric, Genetic, Neonatal, Paediatric and Adult registries.

Whilst there is an increasing number of studies into longer term outcomes, these still remain limited compared to those of early outcomes. The vast majority of these have been reassuring and it appears that an ART singleton born at term and of normal birth weight progresses through childhood normally compared to controls. Little information exists about outcome into later adolescence and adulthood and longer follow up studies are required. Particular areas requiring research are the fertility of adults born by ART and longer term cardiovascular risk.

References

[1] Williams C, Sutcliffe AG, Infant Outcomes of Assisted Reproduction, *Early Hum. Dev.,* 2009;85(11);673-7.

[2] Basatemur E, Sutcliffe AG, Follow Up of Children Born after ART, *Placenta* 2008;29 Suppl. B:135-40.

[3] Johnson M, The Probmematic in-vitro embryo in the age of epigentics, *Reprod. Biomed. Online.* 2005;10 Suppl 1:88-96.

[4] Barker DJ. In utero programming of chronic disease. *Clin. Sci. (Lond)* 1998;95:115-28.

[5] Kallen B, Finnstrom O, Lindam A et al, Trends in delivery and neonatal outcome after in vitro fertilization in Sweeden: data for 25 years *Hum. Reprod.* 2010;25(4):1026-34.

[6] Martin PM, Welch HG, Probabilities for singleton and multiple pregnancies after in vitro fertilistation. *Fertility and Sterility* 1998;70:478-481.

[7] Human Fertilisation and Embryology Authority. Facts and Figure 2006. Fertility Problems and treatment. http://www hfea gov uk/104 html 2008 October 8.

[8] Koivisto M, Jouppila P, Kauppila A, Moilanen I, Ylikorkala O. Twin pregnancy. Neonatal morbidity and mortality. *Acta Obstet. Gynecol. Scand. Suppl.* 1975: 21–9.

[9] Liu C, Blair E. Predicted birthweight for singletons and twins. *Twin Res.* 2002;5:529–37.

[10] Pandian Z, Templeton A, Serour G, Bhattacharya S. Number of embryos for transfer after IVF and ICSI: a Cochrane review. *Hum. Reprod.* 2005;20:2681–7.

[11] Kjellberg AT, Carlsson P, Bergh C. Randomized single versus double embryo transfer: obstetric and paediatric outcome and a cost-effectiveness analysis. *Hum. Reprod.* 2006;21:210–6

[12] Jackson RA, Gibson KA, Wu YW, Croughan MS. Perinatal outcomes in singletons following in vitro fertilization: a meta-analysis. *Obstet. Gynecol.* 2004;103:551–63.

[13] Helmerhorst FM, Perquin DAM, Donker D, Keirse MJNC. Perinatal outcome of 350 singletons and twins after assisted conception: a systematic review of controlled 351 studies. *Br. Med. J.* 2004;328(7434):261–264.

[14] McDonald SD, Han Z, Mulla S et al, Preterm birth and low birth weight among in vitro fertilization singletons: A systematic review and meta-analyses. *Eur. J. Obstet. Gynecol. Reprod. Biol.* 2009;146(2):138-48

[15] Schieve LA, Ferre C, Peterson HB et al. Perinatal outcome among singleton infants conceived through assisted reproductive technology in the United States. *Obstet. Gynecol.* 2004;103(6):1144–53.

[16] Luke B, Brown MB, Grainger DA et al. The effect of early fetal losses on singleton assisted-conception pregnancy outcomes. *Fertil. Steril.* 2009;91(6):2578–85.

[17] Basso O, Baird DD. Infertility and preterm delivery, birthweight, and Caesarean section: a study within the Danish National Birth Cohort. *Hum. Reprod.* 2003;18(11):2478–84.

[18] Zhu JL, Basso O, Obel C, Bille C, Olsen J. Infertility, infertility treatment, and congenital malformations: Danish national birth cohort. *Br. Med. J.;* 2006;333(7570):679.

[19] Ombelet W, Martens G, De Sutter P, et al. Perinatal outcome of 12 021 singleton and 3108 twin births after non-IVF-assisted reproduction: a cohort study. *Hum. Reprod.* April 2006;21(4):1025–32.

[20] De Geyter C, De Geyter M, Steimann S, Zhang H, Holzgreve W. Comparative birth eights of singletons born after assisted reproduction and natural conception in previously infertile women. *Hum. Reprod.* 2006;21(3):705–12.

[21] Romundstad LB, Romundstad PR, Sunde A, et al. Effects of technology or maternal factors on perinatal outcome after assisted fertilisation: a population-based cohort study. *Lancet* 2008;372(9640):737–43.

[22] McDonald SD, Han Z, Mulla S et al, Preterm birth and low birth weight among in vitro fertilization twins: a systematic review and meta-analyses, *Eur. J. Obstet. Gynecol. Reprod. Biol.* 2010: 148(2):105-13.

[23] McDonald S, Murphy K, Beyene J, Ohlsson A. Perinatat outcomes of in vitro fertilization twins: a systematic review and meta-analyses. *Am. J. Obstet. Gynecol.* J2005;193(1):141–52.

[24] Pinborg A, Loft A, Rasmussen S et al, Neonatal outcome in a Danish national cohort of 3438 IVF/ICSI and 10362 non-IVF/ICSI twins born between 1995 and 2000, *Hum. Reprod.* 19(2):435-441

[25] Hansen M, Colvin L, Petterson B, et al. Twins born following assisted reproductive technology: perinatal outcome and admission to hospital. *Hum. Reprod.* 2009: 24(9):2321-31.

[26] Kallen B, Finnstrom O, Lindam A et al, Selected neonatal outcomes in dizygotic twins after IVF versus non-IVF pregnancies. *BJOG* 2010; 117(6) 676-82.

[27] Wennerholm UB, Soderstrom-Anttila V, Bergh C, Children born after cryopreservation of embryos or oocytes: a systematic review of outcome data. *Hum. Reprod.* 2009:;24(9)2158-2172.

[28] Lancaster PAL. Congenital-malformations after in vitro fertilization. *Lancet* 1987;2(8572):1392–3.

[29] Hansen M, Bower C, Milne E, de Klerk N, Kurinczuk JJ. Assisted reproductive technologies and the risk of birth defects — a systematic review. *Hum. Reprod.* 2005;20(2):328–38.

[30] Rimm AA, Katayama AC, Diaz M, Katayama KP. A meta-analysis of controlled studies comparing major malformation rates in IVF and ICSI infants with naturally conceived children. *J. Assist. Reprod. Genet. December* 2004;21(12):437–43.

[31] Reefhuis J, Honein MA, Schieve LA et al. Assisted reproductive technology and major structural birth defects in the United States. *Hum. Reprod.* 2009;24(2):360–6.

[32] Hansen M, Kurinczuk J, Bower C, Webb S, The risk of major birth defects after intracytoplasmic injection and in vitro fertilization, *NEJM* 2002; 346(10):725-730

[33] Olson CK, Keppler-Noreuil KM, Romitti PA, et al. In vitro fertilization is associated with an increase in major birth defects. *Fertil. Steril.* 2005; 84(5):1308–15.

[34] Koivurova S, Hartikainen AL, Gissler M et al, Neonatal outcome and congenital malformations in children born after in-vitro fertilisation, *Hum. Reprod.* 2002; 17(5)1391-1398

[35] Kallen B, Finnstrom O, Lindam A et al, Congenital Malformations in Infants born afterin vitro fertilisation in Sweeden, *Birth Defects Research (Part A)* 2010; 88:137-143.

[36] Klemetti R, Gissler M, Sevon T, et al. Children born after assisted fertilization have an increased rate of major congenital anomalies. *Fertil. Steril.* 2005;84(5):1300–7

[37] Bonduelle M, Wennerholm UB, Loft A, et al. A multi-centre cohort study of the physical health of 5-year-old children conceived after intracytoplasmic sperm injection, in vitro fertilization and natural conception. *Hum. Reprod.* 2005;20(2):413–9.

[38] Ericson A, Kallen B, Congenital Malformations in infants born after IVF: a population based study, *Hum. Reprod.* 2001; 116(3) 504-9.

[39] Rimm AA, Katayama AC, Diaz M, Katayama KP. A meta-analysis of controlled studies comparing major malformation rates in IVF and ICSI infants with naturally conceived children. *J. Assist. Reprod. Genet.* 2004; 21(12):437–43.

[40] Lie RT, Lyngstadaas A, Orstavik KH et al. Birth defects in children conceived by ICSI compared with children conceived by other IVI methods; a meta-analysis. *Int. J. Epidemiol.* 2005;34(3):696–701.

[41] Zhu JL, Basso O, Obel C, Bille C, Olsen J. Infertility, infertility treatment, and congenital malformations: Danish national birth cohort. *Br. Med. J.* 2006;333(7570):679.

[42] Ceelen M, Van Weissenbruch MM, Vermeiden JP, van Leeuwen E, Delemarre-van de Waal HA, Growth and development of children born after in vitro fertilization, *Fertil. Steril.* 2008; 90(5)1662-73.

[43] SutcliffeAG, Peters CJ, Bowdin S, et al. Assisted reproductive therapies and imprinting disorders — a preliminary British survey. *Hum. Reprod.* 2006; 21(4):1009–11.

[44] Lidegaard O, Pinborg A, Andersen AN. Imprinting diseases and IVF: Danish National IVF cohort study. *Hum. Reprod.* 2005; 20(4):950–4.

[45] Wennerholm, U.B., bertsson-Wikland, K., Bergh, C., et al. Postnatal growth and health in children born after cryopreservation as embryos. Lancet 1998; 351, 1085–1090

[46] Brandes, J.M., Scher, A., Itzkovits, J., et al. Growth and development of children conceived by in-vitro fertilization. *Pediatrics* 1992; 90, 424–429.

[47] Knoester, M., Helmerhorst, F.M., Vandenbroucke, J.P., et al.. Perinatal outcome, health, growth, and medical care utilization of 5- to 8-year-old intracytoplasmic sperm injection singletons. *Fertil. Steril.* 2008; 8:1133–1146.

[48] Belva, F., Henriet, S., Liebaers, I., et al. Medical outcome of 8-year-old singleton ICSI children (born > or = 32 weeks' gestation)and a spontaneously conceived comparison group. *Hum. Reprod.* 2007; 22, 506–515.

[49] Basatemur E, Sutcliffe AG Growth of children conceived by IVF and ICSI up to 12 years of age, *Reproductive Biomedicine online* 2010:20;144-149.

[50] Olivennes F, Kerbrat V, Rufat P et al, Follow up of a cohort of 422 children aged 6-13years conceived by in vitro fertilization. *Fertil. Steril.* 1997; 667(2);284-9.

[51] Ludwig AK, Sutcliffe AG, Diedrich K, Ludwig M, Post-neonatal health and development of children born after assisted reproduction: A systematic review of controlled studies, *Eur. J. Obstet. Gynecol. Reprod. Biol.* 2006; 127(1):3-25.

[52] Koivurova, S., Hartikainen, A.L., Sovio, U., et al. Growth, psychomotor development and morbidity up to 3 years of age in children born after IVF. *Hum. Reprod.* 2003; 18, 2328–2336.

[53] Miles, H.L., Hofman, P.L., Peek, J., et al. In-vitro fertilization improves childhood growth and metabolism. *J. Clin. Endocrinol. Metab.* 2007; 92, 3441–3445.

[54] Ceelen M, van Weissenbruch MM, Roos J et al, Body composition in children and adolescents born after in vitro fertilization or spontaneousconception, *J. Clin. Endocrinol. Metab.*, 2007; 92(9) 3417-3423.

[55] Ceelen M, van Weissenbruch MM, Wermeiden JPW et al, Cardiometabolic differences in children born after in vitro fertilization: Follow up study, *J. Clin. Endocrinol. Metab.,* 2008; 93(5); 1682-1688.

[56] Roseboom TJ, van der Muelen JH, Osmond C et al, Coronary heart disease after prenatal exposure to the Dutch famine, 1944-45, *Heart,* 2000; 84(6):595-8.

[57] Ludwig, A.K., Katalinic, A., Thyen, U., et al. Physical health at 5.5 years of age of term-born singletons after intracytoplasmic sperm injection: results of a prospective, controlled, singleblinded study. *Fertil. Steril* 2009; 91:115–124.

[58] Saunders K, Spensley J, Munro J, Halsaz G, Growth and physical outcome of children conceived by in vitro fertilization, *Pediatrics* 1996; 97(5):688-92.

[59] Place I, Englert Y. A prospective longitudinal study of the physical, psychomotor, and intellectual development of singleton children up to 5 years who were conceived by intracytoplasmic sperm injection compared with children conceived spontaneously and by in vitro fertilization. *Fertil. Steril.* 2003; 80:1388–97.

[60] Pinborg A, Loft A, Schmidt L, Anderson AN, Morbidity in a Danish national cohort of 472 IVF/ICSI twins, 1132 non-IVF/ICSI twins and 634 IVF/ICSI singletons: Health related and social implications for the children and their families, *Hum. Reprod.* 2003; 18(6):1234-43.

[61] Leslie GL, Gibson FL, McMahon C et al, Infants conceived using in-vitro fertilization do not over utilize health care resources after the neonatal period, *Human Reprod.* 1998; 13(8):2055-9.

[62] Kallen B, Finnstrom O, Nygren KG, Olausson PO, In vitro fertilization in Sweden: child morbidity including cancer risk, Fertility and Sterility 2005; 84(3):605-10

[63] Ericson A, Nygren KG, Olausson PO, Kallen B, Hospital care utilization of infants born after IVF, *Hum. Reprod.*, 2002; 17(4)929-932.

[64] Koivurova S, Hartikainen AL, Gissler M et al, Post-neonatal hospitalization and health care costs among IVF children: a 7 year follow up study, *Hum. Reprod.* 2007; 22(8)2136-2141.

[65] Klemetti R, Sevon T, Gissler M, Hemminki E, Health of children bon as a result of in vitro fertilization, *Pediatrics* 2006; 118(5)1819-1827.
[66] Hvidtjorn D, Schieve L, Schendel D et al, Cerebral Palsy, Autism Spectrum Disorders and Developmental Delay in Children born after assisted conception, A systematic review and meta-analysisss, *Arch. Pediatr. Adolesc. Med.,* 2009; 163(1): 72-83.
[67] Hvidtjorn D, Grove J, Schendel DE et al, Cerebral palsy among children born after in vitro fertilisation: the role of preterm delivery: a population –based cohort study. *Pediatrics* 2006; 118(2)475-482.
[68] Hvidtjorn D, Grove J, Schendel D et al, Multiplicity and early gestational age contribute to an increased risk of cerebral palsy from assisted conception; a population-based cohort study. *Hum. Reprod.* 2010; 25(8) 2115-23.
[69] Sun Y, Vestergaard M, Christensen J et al. Epilepsy and febrile seizures in children of treated and untreated subfertile couples. *Hum. Reprod.* 2007; 22:215–20.
[70] Stromberg B, Dahlquist G, Ericson A et al. Neurological sequelae in children born after in-vitro fertilisation: a population- based study. *Lancet* 2002; 359:461–5.
[71] Sutcliffe AG, Taylor B, Saunders K et al, Outcome in the second year of life after in vitro fertilization by ICSI: a UK case control study, *Lancet* 2001; 30(357):2080-4.
[72] Koivurova S, Hartikainen AL, Sovio U, et al. Growth, psychomotor development and morbidity up to 3 years of age in children born after IVF. *Hum. Reprod.* 2003; 18:2328–36.
[73] Ponjaert-Kristoffersen I, Bonduelle M, Barnes J et al. International collaborative study of intracytoplasmic sperm injection-conceived, in vitro fertilization-conceived, and naturally conceived 5-year-old child outcomes: cognitive and motor assessments. *Pediatrics* 2005; 115:283–9.
[74] Bowen JR, Gibson FL, Leslie GI, Saunders DM. Medical and developmental outcome at 1 year for children conceived by intracytoplasmic sperm injection. *Lancet* 1998; 351:1529–34.
[75] Knoester M, Helmerhorst FM, Vandenbroucke JP et al, Cognitive development of singletons born after ICSI compared with IVF and natural conception. *Fertil. Steril.* 2008; 90(2)289-96
[76] Banerjee I, Shevlin M, Taranissi M et al. Health of children conceived after preimplantation genetic diagnosis: a preliminary outcome study. *Reprod. Biomed. Online* 2008; 16:376–81.
[77] Nekkebroeck J, Bonduelle M, Desmyttere S, Van den Broeck W, Ponjaert-Kristoffersen I. Mental and psychomotor development of 2-year-old children born after preimplantation genetic diagnosis/screening. *Hum. Reprod.* 2008; 23:1560–6.
[78] Golombok S, Brewaeys A, Cook R et al.The European study of assisted reproduction families: family functioning and child development. *Hum. Reprod.* 1996; 11:2324–31.
[79] Golombok S, Brewaeys A, Giavazzi MT et al. The European study of assisted reproduction families: the transition to adolescence. *Hum. Reprod.* 2002; 17:830–40.
[80] Barnes J, Sutcliffe AG, Kristoffersen I et al. The influence of assisted reproduction on family functioning and children's socio-emotional development: results from a European study. *Hum. Reprod.* 2004; 19:1480–7.
[81] Ponjaert-Kristoffersen I, Tjus T, Nekkerbroeck J et al, Pyschological follow up study of 5 year old ICSI children, *Hum. Reprod.* 200; 19(12)2791-7.

[82] Knoester M, Helmerhorst FM, van der Westerlaken LA et al, Matched follow-up study of 5-8year old ICSI singleotns: child behaviour, parenting stress and child (health related) quality of life, *Hum. Reprod.*, 2007; 22(12)3098-107.

In: In Vitro Fertilization
Editor: Samantha P. Steiger, pp. 83-96
ISBN 978-1-61209-961-3

Chapter IV

Posthumous Sperm Procurement

Sorin Hostiuc,[1] George Cristian Curca,[1] Dan Dermengiu,[1] Florinel Pop,[2] and Mugurel Constantin Rusu[2]
[1]National Institute of Legal Medicine, Bucharest, Carol Davila University of Medicine and Pharmacy, Bucharest
[2]Carol Davila University of Medicine and Pharmacy, Bucharest

Introduction

Posthumous reproduction is defined as the birth of a child after the death of the father; classically it involves a child being conceived before the father's death and being born afterwards. Posthumous assisted reproduction (PAR) is a form of assisted reproductive technology that involves using the reproductive material of a deceased person for procreative purposes[1]; it consists of obtaining spermatozoa from patients which are either death or in a vegetative state (posthumous sperm procurement - PSP), cryopreservation, and the use of advanced assisted reproductive techniques like intracytoplasmic sperm injection (ISCI) for in vitro fertilization.

PAR is usually desired in two situations: (1) when one partner suffers from a potentially fatal illness – the couple stores embryos or gametes with a clear intention of using PAR and (2) urgent sperm retrieval from a man suffering a sudden (usually traumatic) death. The first successful case of PSP was reported by Rothman in 1980[2]; afterwards a few hundred more were reported, more than half being in the US[3].

Legislation in this area is quite summary PSP being a relatively new and not very common method. Most countries don't have a specific legislation in this area (Japan, Ireland, Italy, Singapore, etc.). Other countries completely banned this method (Canada, Denmark, Egypt, France, Germany, Korea, Norway, Spain, Sweden, Netherlands[4, 5] or Romania[6]); in only a few countries like Israel and Australia the method is allowed but only after obtaining a court order. In USA the procedure is not explicitly prohibited, acceptance or prohibition being decided on a case by case basis, usually after a court order. In the UK, according to "Human Fertilization and Embryology Act" the intervention cannot be achieved without written consent from the donors; also the donor is not recognized as the father of the child obtained by this method.

Sperm Harvesting

Postmortem Sperm Viability and Motility

Sperm harvesting can be done on deceased or patients in a perimortem state (brain dead, persistent vegetative state).

It is yet unknown the exact length of postmortem time up until sperm remains viable. In the first reported birth with PSP the postmortem interval was 30 hours[7]; the body was however kept in a refrigerated morgue until the harvest was completed. Without using the refrigerator a few authors gave a 24 hour limit for sperm viability[8] – even if sperm motility was absent the cell membrane was intact. Others stretched that limit to 36 [9], or even 48 hours [10].In perimortem cases it is considered safe to harvest semen for a longer period of time after being declared brain-dead.Songsasen et al, working on mice, found a decrease in sperm motility from 60% in animals dead for up to 12 hours to less than 30% in those dead for 24 hours; viability and acrosome integrity were similar in all groups. The fertilization rate was approximately 6.6% with sperm obtained from mice dead for 24 hours, and 27.3% of the embryos transferred to recipient mice resulted in live births.[11]. Sperm maintains a normal motility and function within the first 3 hours postmortem, after which both motility and viability decrease, at a variable rate (faster for motility), highly dependent on environmental temperature and various pathologies associated with increased postmortem autolysis (infective disorders, MOSF, etc.). In PSP is important to know that sperm cryopreservation will cause further decrease its viability – therefore sperm harvesting should be performed well before the limit for sperm viability is reached.

Ideally sperm harvesting should be realized by an infertility specialist; however, as most cases are associated with traumatic deaths, a specialist is not be readily available – it is possible, in these situations, for an urologist to perform the procedure. Sperm viability and motility should be evaluated for each case.

Sperm Harvesting Methods

Postmortem sperm harvesting is done using different methods, depending on the patient (brain dead or dead) or the physician's experience. Most cited are en-block excision of testis, epididymis and vas deferens with vassal irrigation, orchiectomy and epididymectomy, epididymectomy, testicular extraction, testicular aspiration, testicular fine needle aspiration, testicular percutaneous biopsy, epididymal aspiration, and electroejaculation. Except for the latter, which needs the presence on an intact neurological response, all methods are applicable both to dead and perimortem patients.

Electroejaculation is usually performed using the following method[12]: patient is in lateral decubit position. Bladder is catheterizedbefore the procedure in order to remove the urine and instilled with 5 mL of insemination medium. A rectal probe is inserted with the electrodes facing the anterior direction, towards the ejaculatory organs. The voltage progressively increases until ejaculation is considered to be complete (usually the procedure starts at 4 Volts and ends at 20 Volts)[13]. Anterograde ejaculate is collected into a sterile specimen cup during stimulation; retrograde ejaculate is collected using post-procedure catheterization, in which the bladder is rinsed with another 5 mL of insemination medium. The retrograde portion of the ejaculate is centrifuged at room temperature (5 minutes at 1800 *g*) to yield 1–2 mL of concentrate[13]. Anterograde and retrograde specimens are processed separately using the swim-up procedure or the density gradient method[12]. Prostatic massage can be performed before electroejaculation[13].

Microsurgical epididymal sperm aspiration (MESA): scrotal exploration is conducted through a median raphe incision; under a 10-15x magnification a linear incision of the epididymis tunic is made[14]; individual epididymal tubules are punctured separately with a siliconized glass micropipette attached to an aspiration device (consisting of a 10 cc glass syringe and a 1cc plastic tuberculin syringe), and aspirated[15]. Sequentially more proximal punctures are performed until optimal sperm quality (motility) is obtained[15]. In dead patients motility can be absent; the viability of the spermatozoa must however be checked.

Testicular sperm extraction (TESE): a 250-750 mg of testicular tissue is obtained throughout a biopsy following a single scrotal incision.The biopsy is placed in simulated human tubal fluid (HTF) medium with 6% plasmanate and dispersed in order to isolate individual seminiferous tubules; the obtained suspension is further disrupted by passing it a few times through a 2-gauge angiocatheter. Tissue samples are then analyzed by placing them in a disposable cell-counting chamber and quantifying the presence and number of spermatozoa[16]. An alternative method described by Schlegel involves direct microscopic identification of functioning seminiferous tubules (microdissection TESE); in this method, tunica albugineea is opened widely near its midportion in order to optimize visualization of the testicular parenchyma, which is examined using an operating microscope, at a X20-25 magnification. Larger, more opaque seminiferous tubules within the testicular parenchyma are identified and excised with the surrounding area. Each tissue sample is then further excised to allow the release of spermatozoids from seminiferous tubules. The resulted suspension is analyzed through the technique described above[12,15,17].

*Testicular fine needle aspiration (TFNA):*the scrotal area is cleaned with a clorehexidine solution and draped; multiple punctures are performed in various locations of the testes, using 21-23 gauge butterfly needles, connected to a 20 ml syringe installed on an aspiration handle (Cook) for the application of a steady negative pressure. Following each puncture the needle's content is rinsed in a four-well plate containingHTF-HEPES medium supplemented with 0.4% human serum albumin[18]. The aspirate is centrifuged at 1800 g for 5 minutes; then the re-suspended pellets are layered on a discontinuous Percoll gradient for two layers (47.5 and 95%) and centrifuged at 300g for 20 minutes. The 95% Percoll fraction is transferred in a new tube, washed again using 6 ml HTF-HEPES-albumin medium and re-centrifuged at 1800g for 5 minutes.The final pellet is resuspended in a 50 uU of HTP medium supplemented with 7.5% synthetic serum [18].

*Percutaneous testicular biopsy*is as effective as TESE and as minimally invasive as TFNA. The technique consists in using a large core (14-gauge) biopsy gun with a short, 1 cm excursion. The testis is stabilized between the thumb and the index finger of one hand; the biopsy gun is directed diagonally along the longitudinal axis of the testes, entering the anterior surface of the lower pole, aimed towards the rete testis.[14]. Testicular sperm extraction methods are considered the gold standard in perimortem patients whilst in dead patients en-block excision seems to be the preferred method[19].

Vas deferens irrigation and aspiration. The vas deferens is exposed in the mid-scrotal region and cannulated with a 2-fine gauge iv catheter through a 4 mm longitudinal incision. The vas deferens is irrigated using specific culture medium proximally and distally. The pooled aspirate is prepared using a discontinuous Percoll gradient with exposure to pentoxiphylline and 2-deoxyadenosine, for 30 minutes each.[20].

En-block excision of testes, epididymis and vasa deferens are often preferred in dead patients as they provide a bigger quantity of biologic material, especially useful if PSP is done after more than three hours after death. This is the first method used for PSP, by Rothman in 1980[2]: an incision was made through the prostatic fossa to excise the seminal vesicles, ampullae and pelvic vasa, followed by an inguinal incision to excise the testis and epididymal head.

Sperm Cryopreservation (SC)

PAR Guidelines usually recommend fertilization with posthumous sperm to occur after a period of minimum six months to a year. Therefore IVF techniques using fresh sperm aren't possible, making cryopreservation amandatory step.SC can be done using the classical (slow-freeze) or the vitrification method. Classical method consists of mixing the obtained sperm with a freezing solution containing a cryoprotectant. Most used solutions are hen's egg yolk:citrate buffer 80:20 as the freezing solution and 10% glycerol as cryoprotectant, in equal ratios, at room temperature. Vials are suspended in liquid nitrogen vapors for 15 minutes then inserted in liquid nitrogen at -196 degrees Celsius for long term preservation. In the vitrification method the sperm is initially prepared in a similar fashion as the classical method, but the vials are directly inserted in liquid nitrogen for storage[21]. Recently a new vitrification method, not using cryoprotectanrs was developed; it has the advantage of avoiding the osmotic shock known to be associated with the use of these substances.[22] Recently a new edition of the WHO laboratory manual for the examination and processing of human semen was published[23], containing, in Section 6.2.2 specific guidelines for oligozoospermic samples and surgically retrieved spermatozoa, which can be applied for PSP:

- Semen that contains only a few motile spermatozoa, and sperm suspensions obtained from the genital tract, can be stored for subsequent ICSI;
- If necessary, centrifuge the semen at 1500g for 10 minutes to concentrate the spermatozoa into a minimum volume of about 0.4 ml. Add GEYC and process as described above;
- Epididymal fluid, testicular extracts or other sperm suspensions processed in the laboratory by swim-up or centrifugation on density gradients and resuspended in a sperm preparation medium with HEPES buffer and human serum albumin 4 mg/ml can be cryopreserved with Tyrode's glucose glycerol (TGG) cryoprotectant, or a commercial cryoprotectant containing human albumin.

Modified cryoprotectant (TGG)

1. To 40 ml of sterile Tyrode's solution add 5 ml of sterile human albumin stock (100 mg/ml), 0.9 g of glucose and 5 ml of glycerol;
2. Filter the solution through a 0.45-µm pore filter;
3. Store in 2-ml aliquots at –70 °C.

Procedure

1. If the sample volume is greater than 2.0 ml, and if few motile spermatozoa are present, centrifuge at 1500g for 5 minutes at room temperature;
2. Aspirate the supernatant to leave about 1.0 ml and resuspend the spermatozoa in it. Determine the percentage of motile spermatozoa (PR + NP); if very few motile spermatozoa are present, estimate the number of motile cells under each coverslip;
3. Thaw a 2-ml aliquot of TGG;
4. Add one volume of TGG to one volume of fi nal sperm preparation, gradually, with mixing.[23]

Medical Contraindications

For the IVF technique the contraindications aren't different from other methods; the procedure shouldn't however be performed if:

- The patient has an unknown personal history or an autopsy hasn't been performed[24];
- Death is due to a disease or treatment (especially oncological) known to affect spermatogenesis;
- Genetic disorders affecting either the victim [24] or its immediate relatives;
- HIV, hepatitis or other viral agents are diagnosed; they are known to survive the cryopreservation process[21];
- A positive diagnose for other infective diseases[24];
- Diseases affecting sperm viability are diagnosed.

Bereavement

PSP is usually requested by the spouse in traumatic, violent deaths; we must always keep in mind that a person's judgment is often impaired immediately after the loss of a close person. We, as physicians shouldn't however deny the procedure of sperm retrieval if the law permits it. The obtained biological product can be kept for a long period of time without significantly losing its reproductive capabilities. After such a request however the spouse should undergo a series of medical and psychological consults and discussions, which should encompass all aspects of PSP and subsequent IVF, from medical and financial to psychological and ethical ones. The counselors shouldassess, besides the psychological status of the spouse, its family stability, social and financial support systems[24], etc. Tashconsideres a minimum period of a year should be required beforethe procedure is further carried away[24], a period of time which is considered to be enough for psychological adjustments and bereavement after losing a loved one.

Ethical Issues Regarding PSP

Patients Autonomy. Consent

The fundamental ethical issue in PSP is represented by the patient's autonomy, normally protected throughout the informed consent. Nobody can be constrained to do a medical intervention without its consent, their parents (if under aged) or legal custodians (for persons without decisional capacity). Consent is a dynamic structure during patient-physician interaction – in any moment a new diagnostic procedure may be needed or a new therapeutic line can be open with different costs, risks or benefits. As general elements patient's consent must contain[25]: clinical characteristics of the problem, including those related to diagnostic, therapeutic recommendations, treatment's risks and benefits, intervention costs, alternative procedures if the patient does not agree with the initial version proposed by the doctor and also patient's freedom to accept or refuse treatment.

Usually sperm transfer can be done for the benefit of the couple (to give birth to an heir) or of another person, by donating sperm. Written consent is unnecessary when using sperm to give birth naturally to an heir as mutual agreement is undisputed. In this case reproductive autonomy is not fenced in any way. When usingsperm to give birth to an heir through means of assisted reproductive technologies (ART) usually a written consent in necessary for sperm prelevation (if a medical procedure is needed), analyzis, fertilisation, etc[26-29]. For sperm donation a complete agreement and aknowledgment from the donor is needed. The physician/counsellor must fully disclose all relevant information and must be certain the donor understands it.

A written consent for the purpose of sperm donation must contain at least the following[30]:

- How much time the donated sperm is to be preservated;
- How much time the obtained embryos are to be stored;
- Consent for specific uses of sperm: treatment of others,creating embryos in vitro, the use of those embryos in treatment of others or in research purposes, use of sperm in research purposes;
- Maximum number of families that may have children by usind that donor's sperm;
- Sperm or embryo use if the donor dies or becomes mentally incapacitated; donor can consent to continuos storage of sperm, it's use in treatment of others or in research projects.

Some authors call into question the possibility that dead people have rights as persons [31, 32]. A person may not have fundamental rights related to his being a living person as long as it is not alive. For example, does an Egyptian mummy have the right of self-determination or beneficence? After all it was a person sometimes in the past. If it doesn't, who can determine from when a deceased has or not those fundamental rights? Where to draw the line? A current concept nowadays considers that personhood cannot be taken from a person as long as it lives in the collective memory of other people. Any action directed upon a deceased must take into account his beliefs and wishes as much as possible. For example people are usually reluctant in allowing an autopsy after their own or close one's death. This is maybe the main reason they are not universally done as different studies suggests that autopsies can bringhuge quantities of medical information potentially beneficial to a large number of subjects. If however a benefit can be obtained for that person or its family autopsy is mandatoryin many cases (for example if that person was murdered the prosecutor must order an autopsy to gather prosecutor evidence; if death was sudden, especially in a young age a detailed autopsy might clarify the cause that may affect other family members also[33, 34]).

What about postmortem consent? Besides PSP it has a crucial relevance in organ donation. In organ donation consent can be presumed or informed. Most countries have a policy of informed consent regarding organ donation from the dead – organs are harvested only if that person agrees upon it during his lifetime. Presumed consent, a concept that gathers increased acknowledgment nowadays due to the worldwide organ shortage, means that organ harvesting from a potential donor is done if during his lifetime he didn't sign a document by which refuses to be a donor. Although apparently similar, PSP and cells / tissues / organs donation are not equivalent except through the fact that both involve organic material harvested from a corpse. The purpose is fundamentally different – in the first case to create a life and in a second to save one. Organ donation is an altruistic act while PSP is not. Controlling the fate of their genetic material is a fundamental action and should not be altered in any way. If a person becomes parent after death, without his consent his reproductive autonomy is altered. Let us again take a similar situation from everyday life. A similar breach in reproductive autonomy is found in cases of rape - a breach in woman's reproductive autonomy could lead to an unwanted pregnancy and subsequently to the birth of an undesired child.

In most countries where national legislation allows PSP it is required a previous signed consent from the donor.The question in these cases is how this agreement was achieved and how (if) was documented. Strong[35] describes six hypothetical situations which can happen in these cases. First is the one in which the patient signs (1) or the physician records in a medical document (1b) the donor'sagreement for postmortem sperm harvesting, after a detailed discussion in which all technical, administrative, ethical, legal variables are clarified. In this case the procedure is made by the same physician who obtained the signed consent. The second case is identical with the first except that consent has been obtained by a physician other than the one who will perform the procedure. The third case does not include a physician in decision-making process - the patient signs a notarized document in which it specifies if he allows his own sperm to be harvested after death or persistent vegetative state. The fourth situation is where the patient didn't signed a written consent but there are witnesses, other than his wife who can testify that PSP would have been a valid option for the deceased. The fifth situation is that in which his wife said they've discussed this possibility but there are no other witnesses. The sixth case described by Strong is the one in which the spouses declares that they haven't discussed this possibility but she is certain that her husband would have wanted it. Most authors are agreeing that first two situations have the smallest number of ethical issues regarding consent in PSP. However, neither is completely flawless.

In first scenario there are a few issues that must be addressed. First, this consent is usually signed with some time before his death, when dying wasn't a valid hypothesis for that person. Maybe in the time between signing and death he changed his mind but forgot to revoke the written consent; there are even witnesses who can certify it; what should the physician do? Should he act on the written consent or patient's last requests? Another possible hypothesis would be the one in which the physician knows the patient's views had changed from an informal discussion but the wife still wants to continue with PSP. Should the physician act upon the previous written statement which is the same with patient's legal custodian or upon patient's last wishes? In order to answer to both questions we must clarify the supremacy of a written consent for postmortem issues. Normally a person controls some events happening after its death throughout a will. A will is a signed, notarized statement of a person's wishes concerning the disposal of his property after death (it includes gametes according to EU laws). A will can be modified only by that person and only in writing. Consent on the other hand has more than one form: informed, presumed, free, collective, oral, etc. Consent can be modified after being signed and can be withdrawn is the patient wishes so; this withdrawal can be made by his legal guardian if unable to take this decision by himself.We believe that, if possible, a physician should respect the wishes of the patient, even if not written and even if not with general perception of what is good and what is not, as long as they don't limit other people freedom. If in doubt, the physician must recuse himself as these situations are on the edge of classical bioethics – as with euthanasia a physician cannot be forced to do an act he doesn't consider to do benefits for the patient.

Second, some authors consider that in PSP, as in some other ART's, the physician taking the consent should not be the one who performs the procedure, as conflicts of interest could be raised; some even implied financial or scientific gains could be put on the table which could alter physician's objectivity.

What about the second scenario Strong presents? It doesn't raise conflict of interest issues. It does anyway pose the problem that usually a signed consent is a contract between a patient and a physician. The patient may not accept a certain procedure to be made by another physician. Generally speaking, as Strong outlined, a physician can delegate another person to do a medical procedure – a resident, a nurse, another physician, etc. assuming it was specified in the informed consent[35]. The deceased although doesn't have the option to refuse a certain physician or even a certain procedure as it seems improbable for a written consent to detail these techniqualities.

Third scenario can be seen as a typical will – the deceased wrote down and signed PSP agreement as a last reproductive wish. Different authors suggest this is an atypical consent (considered as a form of substituted judgment and not informed consent as informational flow is unidirectional, from patient to physician) and is regarded with circumspection, its validity being questionable. Strong agrees with this argument and gives as example that in most US Courts consider other similar directives, such as living wills, not to be a proper informed consent. This attitude is unethical from our point of view for two main reasons. First it restrains patient's autonomy: according to Rubin[36] autonomy is the unhindered and independent ability to think, decide and act on a decision, without fear of retaliation; health autonomy is defined by Beauchamp and Childress[37] as self-determination of rights, such as the right to accept or refuse treatment. By not considering a patient's wishes we pose in question his ability to think and decide for himself, which in an ideal world shouldn't happen as long as theresulting act is not interfering with others autonomy. Secondly, by considering the informational flux to be unidirectional we start from the wrong assumption that a physician is the only person capable of giving proper data; nowadays information is widely available through the internet; moreover, many persons suffering from a disease or need for a medical procedure read extensively about it knowing, in many cases, more than many physicians. Let us take another hypothetical example: let's say the person who wants to donate sperm posthumously is the greatest bioethician in PSP in the world; would he need to talk about the technicalities with another physician?

Last two scenarios Strong presents are associating the decision-taking process with the deceased's wife. From his point of view these are not ethically acceptable as they are obvious conflict of interests. The arguments he presents in favor (inferred consent in fifth scenario and substituted judgment in sixth) are not enough to justify sperm retrieval.Moreover in these cases we need to talk about the difference between sperm retrieval from a dying versus death person[38, 39].After White if the husband is in a coma or a persistent vegetative state they are still married; the wife cannot remarry and cannot have a child legally with another man. Also, she still has certain marital rights, including that of reproduction, which would make sperm harvesting permissible. If the husband is dead though, they are not married anymore; the wife is free to marry and legally have children with somebody else, making PSP not permissible with wife's consent alone. What if sperm harvesting is not done for the benefit of the wife but the fiancé's? For example, secondary to a thalamic hemorrhage a 26 year old, unmarried, men became brain-dead. His mother signed the consent for organ harvesting but required also a sperm harvesting procedure for the benefit of his son's fiancé with whom he was engaged for three years and who wanted a child. The application was refused because the parents cannot require sperm harvesting, even in the presence of a written directive from the potential donor. In this case parent's authority as legal guardian's wasn't considered to be enough for sperm harvesting. In this case the law made a clear distinction between wife and fiancé as legal guardian, an attitude which is not completely connected with today's realities in which many couples don't ever get married even if they have children. In some countries artificial insemination and other IVF techniques are permitted to couples living together for at a certain number of years, either married or not. The procedure would have been better denied by arguing specific consent from the donor for sperm insemination was not obtained.

Besides Strong's scenarios another recently emerged case from Israel [40] puts on the table some new ethical issues. KC, an Israeli sergeant was shot by Palestine sniper and dies during hospitalization. The parent requested the physician to retrieve his sperm and preserve it in order for them to find a surrogate mother. After a five year struggle they obtained the right to use their son's sperm for reproductive purposes and also to be acknowledged as grandparents to this child. Even more, there was no written consent from their son, only a videotape in which he stated his wish to have children. In this case gamete property shifted even more from the classical scenarios described by Strong and we think loosens even more the ethical belt strap of PSP; if parents can ask for sperm harvesting from their dead son, what would be next? Strangers could ask for PSP from persons with special characteristics or famous people; then again sperm from famous people could be sold to whoever is interested. Ethical consequences of these acts are unimaginable. This is the reason why we believe that clear guidelines should be drawn in every situation, guidelines with a worldwide availability and acceptance.

Children-Related Ethical Problems

As with other ART, the interests of the child should be an overriding concern for all parties involved. A child born from posthumous sperm is often a child born from grief, out of the natural despair of a person who loses its half. She should know that although ''the desire for posthumous conception is a loving expression in memory of the lost spouse, the offspring has no such memory"[41]. The offspring will be a ''half-orphan'' with subsequent problems: absence of the social father/difference between genetic and social father, doubts about his origin and position in the society, ART-related psychological symptoms [42], issues related to maternal and filial duties [32], etc. There are currently contradictory views about the right of the child born from posthumous sperm to survivor benefits. One might consider that if such rights were granted, the spouse could use this child to access the belongings of the deceased. For example, in Hecht versus Kane, W. Kane left explicit instructions permitting his girlfriend to use his sperm for insemination after he had killed himself. The children from the first marriage sued for nullification to prevent the creation of other contenders to their father's inheritance [43, 44]. On the other side, not permitting a PSP-born child to access survivor benefits/ father's inheritance, especially if informed consent has been given by the father would be discriminative to the child and also considered a breach of father's autonomy. Both the mother and the state must always take the necessary actions for the child to be born as an end by itself and not as a mean to an end.

Guidelines and Recommendations

Ethics Committee of the American Society of Reproductive Medicine

ASRM published a short statement regarding PAR in 2004[45], containing some general recommendations, but avoiding to detail issues like medical-legal problems associated with PAR, or practicing the method without an explicit informed consent [46]. The recommendations were mainly included in four categories – issues regarding the donor, gestating woman, rearing parents and children.

Donor Issues:

- If an individual agrees with PAR, it is totally appropriate to allow it in the absence of any adverse consequences to the living participants for the pregnancy or on the children;
- The gestating woman and the rearing parents should be informed about the procedure and agree with it;
- If donation after death is declined, this should be honored as well;
- A time limit for the procedure after prelevation is not determined; however it should be limited to a few years;
- In case of living donors, if no decision regarding their reproductive samples is obtained, the most likely assumption is that posthumous use is precluded;

- A request from the husband/wife for overriding a prior denial of PAR should be denied;

The gestating woman

- If men want to use frozen embryos or ova for PAR after the death of their spouse, a gestational carrier is needed;
- If the gestational carrier is that men's new wife, she should not be considered a regular surrogate mother;
- If the gestational carrier is not that men's partner she should be considered a traditional surrogate mother, and have all the rights and obligations associated with it.

Rearing parents:

- If they participate in the pregnancy by receiving the embryo as a donation, they should be aware of the deceased status of the donors of gametes/embryos.

Children:

- If the donated gamete is from related individuals the impact is minimal (not significantly different from the one in children born from posthumous birth);
- If the donated gamete is from unreated individuals or deceased for several years the impact is yet undetermined.

ESHRE Task Force on Ethics and Law

The European Society for Human Reproduction and Embriology Task Force on Ethics and Law issued in 2006 a detailed statement regarding PAR[47], focused on the basic bioethical principles; their recommendations have the advantage of addressing various national laws and cultural ideas.

Issues regarding patient autonomy:

- The option for PAR should be offered in the consent form for cryopreservation
- If the clinic refuses the PAR procedure, their informed consent shoud state this option; if patients desire it they should be able to transfer to another clinic willing to realize it;
- An opt-in system is preferred to an opt-out system – in the absence of a written consent no action to obtain reproductive material is to be performed and no use can be made for gametes and embryos;
- Consent should explicitly state the possible use of the cryopreserved gametes for PAR;
- The parents of the deceased or other family members have nothing to say in the matter of PAR;
- The partner can only use the gametes/embryos for their own reproduction; they cannot be donated. The only alternate option is to give them for research purposes;

- The gametes/embryos should be destroyed if both partners die.

*)some members of the Task Force considered PAR outside the family borders to be permissible if a donor consent in that aspect is obtained.

Beneficence:

- Doctors should not assist PAR if a high risk for the children is present;
- There is always a risk for altered psychological development if a child is born and raised without both parents, especially if PAR is done using maternal reproductive material;
- In the period immediately after death of a partner the other often has strong guilt feelings; the surviving partner should not alleviate them using PAR;
- Idealization of the partner.

Justice:

- A child born from PAR shouldn't have fewer rights than a child born throughout other means; therefore is recommended for the child born from PAR to be recognized as the child of the deceased person and it's inheritance rights to be secured;
- In case of embryo/gamete donation to others the general rules of donation apply.

Final recommendations:

- Written consent should be mandatory before the use of the gametes or embryos. Consent should be obtained at the time of storage or before starting the IVF cycle.
- Surviving partner counseling during the decision-making period is needed.
- An embargo period of minimum one year before IVF is needed.

References

[1] Nakhuda, G.S., *Posthumous Assisted Reproduction.Semin. Reprod. Med.*, 2010. 28(04): p. 329,335.

[2] Rothman, C., *A method for obtaining viable sperm in the postmortem state.Fertil. Steril.*1980. 34: p. 512.

[3] Dostal, J., et al., *Post-mortem sperm retrieval in new European Union countries: Case report.Human Reproduction*, 2005. 20(8): p. 2359-2361.

[4] Walker, R. and a. et, *Informed consent to undergo treatment for substance abuse: a recommended approach.Journal of Substance Abuse Treatment*, 2005. 29(4): p. 241-251.

[5] Hurwitz, J.M. and F.R. Batzer, *A guest editorial: Posthumous sperm procurement: Demand and concerns.Obstetrical and Gynecological Survey*, 2004. 59(12): p. 806-808.

[6] Hostiuc, S. (2009) *Tehnici reproductive moderne. Reproducerea asistata.*

[7] Lota, L., *Baby born from dead father's sperm.* Associated Press, 2000.

[8] Spear, K., et al. *Postmortem sperm recovery and preservation: technique and issue for posthumous reproductio.* in *Proceedings of the 69th Annual Meeting of the North Central Section of the American Urological Association.* 1995.

[9] Shefi, S., et al., *Posthumous sperm retrieval: Analysis of time interval to harvest sperm.Human Reproduction,* 2006. 21(11): p. 2890-2893.

[10] Kaabi, M., et al., *Effect of epididymis handling conditions on the quality of ram spermatozoa recovered post-mortem.* Th*eriogenology* 2003. 60: p. 1249 - 1259.

[11] Songsasen, N., J. Tong, and S. Liebo, *Birth of live mice derived by in vitro fertilization with spermatozoa retrieved up to twenty-four hours after death.J. Exp. Zool.,* 1998. 280: p. 189 - 196.

[12] Ohl, D.A., et al., *Electroejaculation and assisted reproductive technologies in the treatment of anejaculatory infertility.Fertility and Sterility,* 2001. 76(6): p. 1249-1255.

[13] Hovav, Y., et al., *Electroejaculation before chemotherapy in adolescents and young men with cancer.Fertility and Sterility,* 2001. 75(4): p. 811-813.

[14] Sheynkin, Y.R., et al., *Controlled comparison of percutaneous and microsurgical sperm retrieval in men with obstructive azoospermia.Human Reproduction,* 1998. 13(11): p. 3086-3089.

[15] Schlegel, P.N., et al., *Epididymal micropuncture with in vitro fertilization and oocyte micromanipulation for the treatment of unreconstructable obstructive azoospermia.Fertility and Sterility,* 1994. 61(5): p. 895-901.

[16] Schlegel, P., et al., *Testicular sperm extraction with intracytoplasmic sperm injection for non-obstructive azoospermia.Urology,* 1997. 49: p. 435 - 440.

[17] Schlegel, P.N., *Testicular sperm extraction: microdissection improves sperm yield with minimal tissue excision.Human Reproduction,* 1999. 14(1): p. 131-135.

[18] Lewin, A., et al., *Delivery following intracytoplasmic injection of mature sperm cells recovered by testicular fine needle aspiration in a case of hypergonadotropic azoospermia due to maturation arrest.Human Reproduction,* 1996. 11(4): p. 769-771.

[19] Land, S. and L.S. Ross, *Posthumous reproduction: Current and future status.* Urologic Clinics of North America, 2002. 29(4): p. 863-871.

[20] Hirsh, A.V., et al., *Case report: Pregnancy using spermatozoa aspirated from the vas deferens in a patient with ejaculatory failure due to spinal injury.Human Reproduction,* 1993. 8(1): p. 89-90.

[21] Chian, R.-C. and P. Queen, *Fertility Cryopreservation,* ed. P.Q. Ri-Cheng Chian. 2010, New York: Cambridge University Press.

[22] Nawroth, F., et al., *Vitrification of human spermatozoa without cryoprotectants.Cryo Letters,* 2002. 23: p. 93 - 102.

[23] *WHO laboratory manual for the Examination and processing of human semen.* 2010, Geneva: WHO.

[24] Tash, J.A., et al., *Postmortem sperm retrieval: The effect of instituting guidelines.Journal of Urology,* 2003. 170(5): p. 1922-1925.

[25] Walker, R., et al., *Informed consent to undergo treatment for substance abuse: a recommended approach.Journal of Substance Abuse Treatment,* 2005. 29(4): p. 241-251.

[26] Crha, I., et al., *Posthumous sperm procurement and use--ethical and legal dilemmas.Ceska Gynekol,* 2004. 69(4): p. 335-9.

[27] Desai, R.V., et al., *Postmortem sperm retrieval: An ethical dilemma.American Journal of Medicine,* 2004. 116(12): p. 858-858.

[28] Hans, J.D., *Attitudes toward posthumous harvesting and reproduction.Death Studies,* 2008. 32(9): p. 837-869.

[29] Miles Rothman, C., *Live sperm, dead bodies.Journal of Andrology*, 1999. 20(4): p. 456-457.

[30] *Consent To The Use And Storage Of Sperm And Embryos In Donation*. 2008, Human Fertilisation and Embriology Authority: UK.

[31] Bahadur, G., *Death and conception.Human Reproduction*, 2002. 17(10): p. 2769-2775.

[32] Batzer, F.R., J.M. Hurwitz, and A. Caplan, *Postmortem parenthood and the need for a protocol with posthumous sperm procurement.Fertility and Sterility*, 2003. 79(6): p. 1263-1269.

[33] Curca, G., et al., *Study on domestic violence: a legal medicine perspective.Romanian Journal of Legal Medicine*, 2008. 16(3): p. 226-242.

[34] Ciobanu, M., et al., *Sudden death in pregnancy with HIV.Romanian Journal of Legal Medicine*, 2007. 15(3): p. 195-201.

[35] Strong, C., *Gamete retrieval after death or irreversible unconsciousness: What counts as informed consent?* Cambridge Quarterly of Healthcare Ethics, 2006. 15(2): p. 161-171.

[36] Rubin, S., *When Doctors Say No: The Battleground of Medical Futility*. 1998, Bloomington: Indiana University Press.

[37] Beauchamp, T. and J. Childress, *Principles of Biomedical Ethics*. 2001, Oxford: Oxford University Press.

[38] Orr, R.D. and M. Siegler, *Is posthumous semen retrieval ethically permissible?J. Med. Ethics,* 2002. 28(5): p. 299-302.

[39] White, G., *Commentary: Legal and ethical aspects of sperm retrieval.Journal of Law, Medicine and Ethics,* 1999. 27: p. 359-361.

[40] Landau, R., *Posthumous sperm retrieval for the purpose of later insemination or IVF in Israel: An ethical and psychosocial critique.Human Reproduction*, 2004. 19(9): p. 1952-1956.

[41] Corrigan, E., S.E. Mumford, and M.G.R. Hull, *Posthumous storage and use of sperm and embryos: Survey of opinion of treatment centres.British Medical Journal*, 1996. 313(7048): p. 24.

[42] McWhinnie, A.M., *Children From Assisted Reproductive Technology: The Psychological Issues and Ethical Dilemmas.Early Child Development and Care*, 2000. 163(1): p. 13 - 23.

[43] *Hecht v. Superior Court (Kane).* West's California reporter, 1996. 59: p. 222-229.

[44] Collins, J.L., *Hecht v. Superior Court: recognizing a property right in reproductive material.* University of Louisville *journal of family law* / University of Louisville School of Law, 1994. 33(3): p. 661-684.

[45] *Posthumous reproduction.* Fertility and Sterility, 2004. 82(Supplement 1): p. 260-262.

[46] Nakhuda, G.S., *Posthumous assisted reproduction.Seminars in Reproductive Medicine,* 2010. 28(4): p. 329-335.

[47] Ethics, E.T.F.o., et al., *ESHRE Task Force on Ethics and Law 11: Posthumous assisted reproduction.Human Reproduction*. 21(12): p. 3050-3053.

In: In Vitro Fertilization
Editor: Samantha P. Steiger, pp. 97-107
ISBN 978-1-61209-961-3

Chapter V

Assisted Reproductive Technologies for Serodiscordant Couples with an HIV-1 Infection

Andrea Giannotti Galuppo[1*] ***and Roseli Fernandes Gonçalves***[2†]
[1]Embryology and Animal Reproduction Biotech Laboratory, College of Veterinary Medicine, Rio Grande do Sul Federal University, Porto Alegre, RS, Brazil
[2]Department of Animal Reproduction, College of Veterinary Medicine and Animal Sciences, São Paulo University, São Paulo, SP, Brazil

Abstract

The use of assisted reproductive technologies (ART) has been increasing over the past three decades. In developed countries ART account for 1–3% of annual births. The ART developments allow several applications over infertility, for example, serodiscordant human immunodeficiency virus-1 (HIV-1) couples. Many HIV-1 positive people of reproductive age are getting married and wish to have children safely. The use of ART apparently is a viable and safe solution to this problem. This review aims to summarize the current state of the art of assisted reproductive technologies for serodicordant couples with an HIV-1 infection. As fertility care for HIV-1 infected couples is complex it is important to analyze some points. In the 1980s until late 1990s life expectancy after HIV-1 diagnosis was around 20 months, because of such a short life expectancy patients were advised not to get pregnant. Couples with one HIV-1 infected partner had a high risk of horizontal and vertical transmission of the virus, and as consequence they were advised to always use condoms, and if a pregnancy occurs an abortion was indicated. Also it is important to consider the very low sensitivity and a chance of false-negative result of the test available to detect the virus. However, since the application of highly active antiretroviral therapy (HAART), people infected with HIV-1 have been living longer. And in the situation of serodiscordant couples a large body of evidence has demonstrated that the use of assisted reproductive technology, as IUI, IVF and ICSI is effective for active pregnancy, while eliminating the risk of viral

* Telephone: 55 - 51 - 33086126; Fax: 55 - 51 -33087305.
† Telephone: 55 - 11- 30917914; Fax: 55 - 11 - 30917412.

transmission. Furthermore, far more sensitive polymerase chain reaction-based methods to detect the presence of HIV-1 not only in blood but also in other fluids including semen had become available. In this review those points will be analyzed with the intent of contributing for a better understanding of this question in order to offer up-to-date assisted reproductive support.

1. Introduction

The use of assisted reproductive technologies (ART) has been increasing over the past three decades. The ART developments allow several applications over infertility, for example, serodiscordant human immunodeficiency virus-1 (HIV-1) couples. Many HIV-1 positive people in reproductive age are getting married and wish to have children safely (Bujan et al., 2007). According to the World Health Organization HIV-1 affects ~40 million persons around the world (UNAIDS/WHO, 2008). Considering that sexual activity is the principal mode of transmission, the use of ART apparently is a viable and safe solution to this problem.

However, in the 1980s until late 1990s life expectancy after HIV-1 diagnosis was around 20 months (van Leeuwen et al., 2009). Because of such a short life expectancy patients were advised not to get pregnant (van Leeuwen et al., 2009). The American Society for Reproductive Medicine (ASRM) and the Center for Disease Control (CDC) considered HIV-1 infection to be a contraindication for ART (Sauer, 2003; Bertrant et al., 2004).

Nevertheless, since the mid-1990s, the use of highly active antiretroviral therapy (HAART) has spread and the AIDS mortality rate has decrease by more than 80% in the industrialized world (Kato et al., 2006). The effects of HAART on blood viral load are now well known and this treatment significantly reduces viral load in blood and seminal plasma (Bujan et al., 2007). As a result of HAART, the general health and life expectancy of HIV-1 seropositive patient is much improved (Peña et al., 2002; Sauer, 2003; Kashima et al., 2009).

According to Nicopoullus et al. (2004) because patients have an estimated life expectancy of at least 20 years from diagnosis, it has become no longer justifiable to deny fertility treatment to HIV-positive adults of whom 75% are between 20 and 40 years of age. The improvement in the quality of life and the increase in the assymptomatic period of infected persons have given many the hopes of starting a family and living a “normal life” (Kato et al., 2006; van Leeuwen et al., 2009). Therefore, this review aims to summarize the current state of the art of ART for serodicordant couples with an HIV-1 infection.

2. Natural Conception, Semen from a HIV-Negative Donor and ART

Being infected by HIV-1 does not preclude being infertile (ASRM, 2010). However, couples with one HIV-1 infected partner had a high risk of horizontal and vertical transmission of the virus, as consequence they were advised to always use condoms, and, if a pregnancy occurs, an abortion was indicated (Nicopoullos et al, 2004). Nevertheless even knowing that abandonment of safe-sex practices would lead to HIV-1 infections in some healthy women attempting pregnancy it cannot be condoned (Sauer, 2003).

Nicopoullos et al (2004) reported that in a serodiscordant couple, the woman has a 0.1% to 0.2% risk of acquiring HIV per act of unprotected intercourse, so attempting to conceive naturally carries a serious risk to the uninfected woman and child. For couples who desire a child, this risk severely limits their reproductive options (Peña et al., 2002; van Leeuwen et al., 2009). The consideration of adoption, the refraining from having children or artificial insemination with semen from an HIV-negative donor remains the safeties alternatives. But, patients are often reluctant to accept those alternatives particularly if they have an otherwise normal reproductive ability (Peña et al., 2002). Considering that, reproductive assistance to HIV-discordant couples can make a significant impact in prevention of viral transmission (Nicopoullos et al, 2004).

Nakuda et al. (2005) showed in a survey of 1440 patients with HIV that 29% expressed desire for children, and many serodiscordant couples reject the notion of using donor sperm for conception. The patients may reject those options and prefer to use the husband's processed sperm despite the potential risk of infection, because they strongly desire to have their own biological children (Peña et al., 2002; Peña et al., 2003; Sauer, 2003). That corroborates Van Leeuwen et al (2009) observation that in the situation of serodiscordant couples a large body of evidence has demonstrated that the use of ART, as intrauterine insemination (IUI), in vitro fertilization (IVF) and intracytoplasmic sperm injection (ICSI) is effective for active pregnancy, while eliminating the risk of viral transmission.

3. Assisted Reproductive Technology (ART)

As exposed by van Leeuwen et al. (2009) as fertility care for HIV-1-infected couples is complex, it is crucial that HIV physicians, reproductive gynecologists, reproductive biologists and virologists work together on the fertility treatment of HIV-1-infected patients and extend their knowledge on reproductive issues, in order to offer these couples up-to-date ART support. Nakuda et al. (2005) mention that with ART development especially for use of serodiscordant couples the American College of Obstetrics and Gynecology and the ASRM endorse the use of those technologies for men, women and couples infected with HIV-1. The ASRM (2010) showed no significant differences in clinical pregnancy rates between HIV-1 infected infertile patients and seronegative-matched controls. Appropriately counseled couples who wish to safely conceive now have an alternative to natural conception and its attendant transmission risk (Peña et al., 2002). However, it was also understood that the procedure was not risk free and carried with it a small undefined possibility for infection (Sauer, 2003).

3.1. Assisted Reproductive Technology in Seropositive Women

Several reports have questioned the quality of spontaneous fertility in HIV-positive women (Hinz et al., 2002; Terriou et al., 2005). The right to be treated is questioned in cases of seropositive women where the viral process is an advanced stage (Marina et al, 1998).

Terriou et al (2005) described that women with HIV infection appear to have a higher incidence of gynecological complications, anovulation and early menopause, and to experience more difficulty in becoming pregnant.

An important factor in denying care to HIV-1 infected women is the need of HAART suspention during the first 3 months of pregnancy owing to its possible teratogenic effects (Marina et al., 1998). Additionally, another important factor relates to concerns of viral contamination of tissue cultures or storage facilities within the IVF-laboratory setting. Aspiration of eggs for in vitro fertilization is not bloodless procedure (Sauer, 2003).

According to Melo et al. (2008) it is unknown whether the HIV-1 presence would lead to abnormal embryo development and/or a decline in the pregnancy rate. In a report presented by ASRM (2010) in 52 HIV-female serodiscordant couples, there were no significant differences for number of mature oocyte per oocytes retrieval, implantation rate, or clinical pregnancy rate compared with controls. However, the fertilization rate for HIV-female serodiscordant couples was lower than that for controls. Terriou et al. (2005) reported that pregnancy is less frequent in HIV-positive women than uninfected women exposed to the same risk of pregnancy. Baccetti et al (1998) exposed unfertilized human oocytes partly surrounded by follicular cells to low doses of HIV-1 and found that they remained negative for the presence of HIV-1 DNA suggesting the resistance of oocytes to HIV-1 penetration, possibly as a result of the absence of specific receptors for the virus as assessed by immunocytochemestry. Terriou et al. (2005) reported that the only parameters suggestive of hypofertility in HIV-1 infected patients in comparison with seronegative controls was the increase in cancellation rate (15.2 versus 4.9%, $p<0.001$) and the duration of ovarian stimulation (13.3 versus 11.7% days, $p<0.01$).

There has been considerable discussion in the recent literature about the expansion of infertility treatment to include human immunodeficiency virus (HIV) positive women (Nahvi et al., 2001; Sauer 2003; Terriou et al., 2005). Since 2001, French law has allowed assisted reproduction teams to treat HIV-1 infected women under strict conditions: absence of current pathology, CD4(+) counts $>200mm^3$, and stable HIV-1 RNA level. Regarding HIV-1 RNA level, the law stipulates that assisted reproduction protocols must be cancelled if HIV-1 RNA increase is >0.5 log between 4 months before the demand and inclusion and between two trimester blood analysis during the protocol (Terriou et al., 2005). However according to Sauer (2003) women were required to be HIV-1 seronegative. It was elected not to offer treatment to HIV-1 seropositive women, because vertical transmission is known to occur in the fetus. Sauer (2003) argued that vertical transmission to the unborn fetus justifies the exclusion of seropositive women from active intervention with invasive methods such as IVF.

3.2. Assisted Reproductive Technology in Seropositive Men

It has not been determined whether HIV is attached to spermatozoa or whether spermatozoa can be infected with HIV (Kato et al., 2006). Some studies have indicated that HIV can bind and enter into spermatozoa (Baccetti et al., 1998; Kato et al., 2006). Nevertheless, other authors have detected HIV-1 only in seminal plasma and/or in the HIV-1 target cells present in the ejaculate (lymphocytes and macrophages), but not in gametes (Sauer, 2003; Garrido et al., 2006; Kashima et al., 2009). The presence of HIV-1 in spermatogonia, spermatocytes and to a lesser degree in spermatids has been demonstrated

(Marina et al., 1998). Nicopoullos et al. (2004) reported that the virus is present in semen as free virus in seminal plasma, and as cell-associated virus in the nonsperm cells, but there is little evidence to support HIV being able to attach to or infect sperm.

A question that immediately arose after the convincing demonstration of the presence of HIV-1 in spermatozoa was the viability of infected sperm cells and their implication in fertilization processes (Baccetti et al., 1998). Fatehi et al. (2006) studied the possible negative effect on the sperm of a seropositive man on the fertilization of oocytes and early embryonic development. They described that sperm DNA damage would affect sperm physiology and it would affect embryo development at the stage that the embryo genome (including the paternal damaged DNA) expression is initiated. A recent study showed that fertilization and cleavage rate were lower for HIV-male serodiscordant couples than that for controls (ASRM, 2010). However a study performed by Melo et al. (2008) presented a similar ability to implant of embryos produced from sperm obtained from HIV-1-infected males when compared with a control group formed by women with tubal occlusion undergoing ICSI.

Another factor of research interest, considering seropositive men, is the correlation between HIV-1 infection and semen parameters, blood CD4 levels and viral load levels. Receiving HAART seems not to impair spermatogenesis in HIV-seropositive males (Garrido et al, 2005). Garrido et al. (2005) demonstrated that as the disease evolves in time, sperm motility is not impaired. Garrido et al. (2006) presented that there are data to demonstrate that the level of infection, general health, and antiretroviral treatments do not greatly influence sperm parameters. However Melo et al. (2008) reported that the immunologic condition and age aggressive treatments received by HIV-positive males could interfere with sperm function. The impairment in sperm production or quality could be caused by their long-time exposure to HAART (Melo et al., 2008).

Nakuda et al. (2005) suggests that viral load (HIV-RNA-PCR) was required to be less than 30,000 copies per milliliter, and stable over 6 months, CD4+ T-cell counts also must have demonstrated stability, over the 6 months prior to treatment. Female partners were required to demonstrate HIV-1 seronegativity. A general health and reproductive screening was performed on couples prior to attempting ART, including serological testing for hepatitis.

Nicopoullos et al (2004) reported that the perspective is now supported by reports of over 300 healthy children born after more than 2300 cycles of sperm washing (and viral-detection testing) and IUI or IVF/ICSI worldwide, with no reported seroconversions in either partner or children. HIV-1-seropositive men were required to be in good health, without active AIDS-defining illness, verified by a letter of clearance from their infectious disease specialist (Nakuda et al., 2005).

3.3. How to Remove HIV-1 from Infected Semen

Given the prevalence of the HIV-1 it is important to develop methods with the aim of how to remove HIV from infected semen samples to prevent vertical transmission of the disease in assisted reproductive medicine (Morozumi et al., 2004). Therefore, it would be possible for an HIV-infected man to father children without risk of viral transmission, if HIV-free spermatozoa can be obtained from his semen (Kato et al., 2006). The implementation of sperm-preparation techniques, popularly referred to as "sperm washing", appears to reduce the probability of horizontal transmission and has been recommended as a means for HIV-1 serodiscordant couples to have a child (Sauer, 2003). According to Fiore et al. (2005) in serodiscordant couples with the male infected, sperm wash has been demonstrated to be the most effective procedure to reduce semen HIV-1 load. The clinical value of sperm washing as well as its risks was first reported by Semprini and Levi-Setti (1992), and since then, it has been confirmed by many authors examining both methodological issues and clinical data (Nahvi et al., 2001; Kato et al., 2006; Kashima et al., 2009).

Semprini and Levi-Setti (1992) reported that in their program couples conceived after 1-5 insemination attempts, and in 59% of cases the first attempt proved successful. Recent evidence shows that swim up processing of semen reduces HIV-1 seminal viral load to undetectable levels (Nahvi et al., 2001). Kato et al. (2006) showed that spermatozoa collected by the swim-up method were neither infected with HIV-1 nor had HIV-1 attached to them. Percoll-density gradient centrifugation and swim-up of motile spermatozoa are also employed and the spermatozoa suspension obtained is tested for the presence of HIV-RNA (Fiore et al., 2005). Hanabusa et al. (2000) showed that swim-up processing after Percoll gradient centrifugation of the infected semen reduced the HIV-1 RNA and HIV-1 proviral DNA to undetectable levels.

Apparently conventional sperm separation wash techniques will reduce HIV-1 RNA levels to undetectable in a majority of cases (Anderson and Politch, 2003). Marina et al. (1998) reported a pregnancy following ICSI from an HIV-1 positive man. After the semen washing they performed a PCR for detecting HIV-RNA and DNA and they observed a negative result on the remaining spermatozoa. Since most HIV RNA transcripts are associated with noninfectious virus particles and documented titers of infectious HIV-1 particles in semen are considerably lower than RNA copy number (range: 0 to 100), low levels of residual HIV-1 RNA in the inseminating fraction are probably clinically insignificant (Anderson and Politch, 2003).

Nevertheless, its efficiency is not absolute. It is not clear yet if the efficacy of sperm wash depends on the viral load of the ejaculate, on the laboratory handling, or on both (Melo et al., 2008). Sperm parameters are not significantly different from those that the World Health Organization considers to be normal. Fiore et al (2005) described that previous reports have claimed that sperm washing is able to entirely remove the virus in all semen samples tested, regardless of the amount of virus present in the sample. However Garrido et al. (2005) reported that they were unable to detect a parameter that could help in the prediction of the sperm wash results, which remained positive in 10% of the samples. Marina et al. (1998) published an incidence of viral presence after wash in >5% of the samples. Garrido et al. (2002) because of the assay's detection limit reported an increase of 12% positive samples after wash.

3.4. Intrauterine Insemination (IUI), in Vitro Fertilization (IVF) and Intracytoplasmic Sperm Injection (ICSI)

In 1992, Semprini and Levi-Setti were the first to report the results of an insemination program using spermatozoa obtained after specific sperm preparation, allowing serodiscordant couples with an HIV-1 infected male partner to have a child while reducing the risk of transmission to the woman (Semprini and Levi-Setti, 1992; Bujan et al., 2007). In the last decade IUI of washed sperm from HIV-positive men has emerged as a potentially safe means of assisting serodiscordant couples in conceiving children while substantially reducing the risk of HIV-1 transmission (Peña et al., 2003). Semprini and Levi-Setti (1992) suggested that limiting fertilization attempts (ideally to a single one) by ovarian hyperstimulation reduces the chances of infection by about 50-fold, even if processed semen still contains HIV. But, according to Van Leeuwen et al. (2009) it is therefore important to identify prognostic factors for IUI outcome, and to adjust assisted reproductive technology protocols.

However it is important to remark that there are some cases in which IUI is not indicated: woman with obstructed Fallopian tubes, cases of low-quality semen and faulty IUI methods. In order to achieve higher pregnancy rates the sperm washing must be performed, but the man must have a sufficient quantity of spermatozoa in the ejaculate (Bujan et al., 2007). However to achieve higher virus elimination rates, the number of collected spermatozoa becomes small (Kato et al., 2006). In these cases, intracytoplasmic sperm injection (ICSI) or in vitro fertilization (IVF) must be performed.

Considering that some teams have proposed IVF-ICSI as the method of choice for serodiscordant couples (Peña et al., 2003; Sauer, 2003; Nicopoullos et al, 2004; Kato et al., 2006; Bujan et al., 2007; Kashima et al., 2009). Peña et al. (2002) report the first live births of two uninfected children from consecutive pregnancies in an HIV-serodiscordant couple who conceive through IVF-ICSI and ET. Melo et al. (2008) showed that the embryo quality and ICSI outcome are not affected by HIV-1 infection in serodiscordants couples with infected males. Marina et al. (1998) described that the ICSI technique involves using only one spermatozoon per oocyte and it would therefore seem logical that risk of infection is lower than in IUI, where woman receive millions of spermatozoa. Peña et al. (2003) and Sauer (2003) described that ICSI reduces the inoculums of HIV particles, if indeed present in motile sperm, by a factor of 10^6, as an oocyte is now exposed to only a single sperm. Those authors showed also that IVF-ICSI using processed semen in HIV-1 seropositive male discordant couples to be safe without a documented conversion.

Table 1. Results of ART in HIV-1-discordant couples with infected male partner

Reference	Couple	Cycle	Pregnancy
IUI treatment			
Semprini et al. (1997)	350	1000	200 (20)
Marina et al. (1998)	63	101	31 (30.7)
Weigel et al (2001)	47	101	15 (14.9)
Bujan et al. (2004)	56	213	37 (17.4)
Nicopoullus et al. (2004)	105	133	25 (18.8)
Savasi et al. (2007)	581	2400	456 (19.6)
IVF or ICSI treatment		Embryo transfer	
Weigel et al. (2001)	19	31	15 (48.4)
Sauer et al. (2002)	34	55	25 (45.5)
Pena et al. (2003)	61	100	35 (35)
Ohl et al. (2003)	47	41	20 (48.8)
Chu et al. (2005)	92	146	54 (37)
Savasi et al. (2007)	160	278	65 (23)
Kashima et al. (2009)	27	33	22 (60.6)

ART, assisted reproduction technique; IUI, intrauterine insemination. (Kashima et al., 2009).

Nicopoullos et al. (2004) recommend that couples arrange for sperm washing of a semen sample in advance, with cryopreservation if no HIV RNA is detected to act as backup. Selecting a single sperm from a sample containing thousands of sperm that have tested negative for HIV-1 RNA provides additional insurance that the inseminating sperm will be HIV-1 negative (Anderson and Politch, 2003). Garrido et al. (2002) and Kato et al. (2006) emphasize that in IVF or ICSI, it is possible to confirm the absence of HIV-1 in the culture medium of fertilized eggs before embryo transfer and the IVF or ICSI procedures could be conducted using frozen spermatozoa that had been confirmed negative for HIV-1. Kashima et al. (2009) also report an advantage of IVF or ICSI over IUI related to the increase in pregnancy rates per treatment cycle (table 1). IVF or ICSI should decrease the number of attempts needed to establish a successful pregnancy, thus further reducing potential viral exposure from repetitive treatment cycles (Kashima et al., 2009). Anderson and Politch (2003) described similar results related to ICSI pregnancy rates per cycle in HIV-1 discordant couples that are about twice that of IUI rates.

However a serious caveat to recommending ICSI as the method of choice for HIV-1 discordant couples is the requirement of a sophisticated assisted reproduction technology facility and the high cost of the procedure (Anderson and Politch, 2003). Sauer (2003) reported that the average price of a single attempt at IVF-ICSI with medications is almost four times the cost of an IUI then the IUI with washed sperm represents a much cheaper alternative. However, the IUI is less efficacious than IVF-ICSI and typically requires multiple treatment cycles – and, thus, multiple exposures to virus – in order to demonstrate comparable success rates. Thus, for many choosing IUI the overall cost of care might not be appreciable cheaper, while the cumulative risks might be greater (Sauer, 2003).

4. Laboratory Quality Control Assurance

It was feared that HIV-1 posed an unacceptable danger to laboratory personnel performing assisted reproductive techniques. It was also believed that bringing HIV-1 into the IVF laboratory could possibly cross-contaminated other patients' samples in tissue culture, which threatens the well-being of other couples undergoing therapy within the same center (Sauer, 2003). The viral risk area was dedicated purely to these biological samples, including a biosafety cabinet workstation, an exclusive centrifuge with anti-aerosol lids, and a nitrogen tank solely for storage of these potentially infectious samples. And the working area is disinfected extensively after each protocol, thus eliminating any possible cross-contamination (Garrido et al, 2005; Nakuda et al., 2005).

As a control method the nested polymerase chain reaction (nPCR) has been routinely used. Van Leeuwen et al. (2009) reported that far more sensitive PCR-based methods to detect the presence of HIV-1 not only in blood but also in other fluids including semen had become available. According to Garrido et al. (2005, 2006) several methodologies have been used for detecting HIV in sperm, although nPCR has been demonstrated to be the most sensitive, because it is effective in detecting a single viral RNA or DNA particle. Therefore considering that sperm-washing procedures can eliminate the virus from sperm, a subsequent nPCR determination confirms their absence, so that the sperm may be used in ART with a negligible risk of transmission (Garrido et al., 2006).

Garrido et al (2005) described the importance of correct laboratory manipulation. Considering that a positive result could be a consequence of incorrect laboratory manipulation. According to them the modus operandi in the laboratory must be focused on two aspects: first, to eliminate any viral particle, since nPCR is an extremely sensitive method, and any viral residue will be detected thus yielding a positive result and forcing the discard of the sample. Secondly, optimize the sperm washing procedure to ensure that as many motile sperm as possible was kept, to permit as many ICSI procedures as possible. Then, if the manipulation in the laboratory is relevant for the results, this is a delicate equilibrium that sometimes can be broken, therefore producing a positive result (Garrido et al., 2005).

Another use for that technique is the control of seroconversion on pregnant and nonpregnant women after embryo transfer. HIV-RNA-PCR was performed on pregnant women every 3 months during the pregnancy. Infants and mothers were tested by either 6 months HIV-RNA-PCR or HIV-DNA-PCR at birth and 3 and 6 months later. In nonpregnant patients, HIV-EIA screens were performed 3 months after embryo transfer. Patients must be contacted annually thereafter for additional follow-up (Nakuda et al., 2005).

Conclusions

Treatment of patients with HIV-1 infection remains one of the most difficult challenges of our time (Sauer, 2003). The virus is viewed as a modern plague, presenting a formidable challenge to society and medicine (Sauer, 2003). The detection of HIV-1 RNA in cells and the reliability of the tests performed are a matter for discussion with the virologists (Bujan et al., 2007). A better understanding of the biology of the virus and its mode of transmission has led to remarkable therapeutic advances and altered the clinical course of illness (Sauer, 2003).

The use of HAART has extended the life expectancy of most patients indefinitely. Physicians now consider HIV to be a “chronic illness” rather than a deadly disease. Emphasis on living a ‘normal’ productive life is an important part of the psychosocial orientation of all individuals harboring HIV-1 virus. However, the inability to begin a family threatens the ability of HIV-1 seropositive individuals to achieve one of life’s most celebrated milestones (Sauer, 2003). However offering assisted reproduction to HIV positive individuals remains controversial (Nakuda et al., 2005).

A decade ago, HIV-1 serodiscordant couples were not routinely considered candidates for reproductive care (Peña et al., 2002). However, a permissive attitude toward providing reproductive care to HIV-1 seropositive patients recognizes the autonomy of infected individuals, some of whom would assume risks to attempt to conceive naturally in the absence of reproductive assistance(Nakuda et al., 2005). These individuals are actively making plans for a future which logically includes establishing long-term relationships and beginning a family (Sauer, 2003).

Advances in ART (such as sperm washing techniques and IVF-ICSI), coupled with the improvements in HIV care, now permit couples to raise a family and remain healthy (Peña et al., 2002; Anderson and Politch, 2003). The cumulative data strongly suggests that ART is effective and safe for HIV-discordant couples and may provide considerable risk reduction of viral transmission (Nakuda et al., 2005).

References

American Society for Reproductive Medicine HIV-1 or hepatitis C chronic infection in serodiscordant infertile couples has no impact on infertility treatment outcome. *Fertility and Sterility,* 93 (3): 1020-1023, 2010.

Anderson D.J., Politch J.A. Providing fertility care to HIV-1 serodiscordant couples: a biologist's point of view. *The American Journal of Bioethics*, 3 (1): 47-49, 2003.

Baccetti B., Benedetto A., Collodel G., di Caro A., Garbuglia A.R., Plomboni P. The debate on the presence of HIV-1 in human gametes. *Journal of Reproductive Immunology*, 41: 41-47, 1998

Bertrand E., Zissis G., Marissens D., Gerard M., Rozenberg S., Barlow P., Delvigne A. Presence of HIV-1 follicular fluids, flushes and cumulus oophorus cell of HIV-1-seropositive women during assisted-reproduction technology. *AIDS,* 18 (5): 823-825, 2004.

Bujan L., Dandin M., Moinard N., Plante P., Parinoud J., Pasquier C. Azoospermic HIV-1 infected patients wishing to have children: proposedstrategy to reduce HIV-1 transmission risk during sperm retrieval and intracytoplasmic sperm injection: case report. *Human Reproduction*, 22(9): 2377-2381, 2007

Fatehi AN, Bevers MM, Schoevers F, Roelen BA, Colenbrander B, Gadella BM. DNA damage in bovine sperm does not block fertilization and early embryonic development but induces apoptosis after the first cleavages. *Journal of Andrology*, 27:176–88, 2006.

Fiore J.R., Lorusso F., Vacca M., Ladisa N., Greco P., De Palo R. The efficiency of sperm washing in removing human immunodeficiency virus type 1 varies according to the seminal viral load. *Fertlity and Sterility*, 84 (1): 232-234, 2005.

Garrido N., Mesenger M., Belver J. In vitro fertilization with intracytoplasmic sperm injection for human immunodeficiency virus-1 serodiscordant couples. *American Journal of Obstetrics and Gynecology*, 187 (1): 1121, 2002.

Garrido N., Mesenguer M., Remohí J., Simón C., Pellicer A. Semen characteristics in human immunodeficiency vírus (HIV) and hepatitis C (HCV) seropositive males: predictors of the success of viral removal after sperm washing. *Human Reproduction*, 20 (4): 1028-1034, 2005.

GarridoN., Remohi J., Mesenquer M. The effectiveness of modified sperm washes in severely oligoasthenozoospermic men infected with human immunodeficiency and hepatitis C viruses. *Fertility and Sterility*, 86(5): 1544-1546, 2006.

Hanabusa H., Kuji N., Kato S., Tagami H., Kaneko S., Tanaka H., Yoshimura Y. An evaluation of semen processing methods for eliminating HIV-1. *AIDS*, 14: 1611-1616, 2000.

Hinz S, McCormack D and van der Spuy ZM. Endocrine function in HIV-infected women. *Gynecology and Endocrinology*, 16: 33–38, 2002.

Kashima K., Takakuwa K., Suzuki M., Makino M., Kaneko S., Kato S., Hanabusa H., Tanaka K. Studies of assisted reproduction techniques (ART) for HIV-1-discordant couples using washed sperm and the nested PCR method: a comparison of the pregnancy rates in HIV-1-discordant couples and control couples. *Japanese Journal of Infectious Diseases*, 62: 173-176, 2009.

Kato S., Hanabusa H., Kaneko S., Takakuwa K., Suzuki M., Kuji N., Jinno M., Tanaka R., Kojima K., Iwashita M., Yoshimura Y., Tanaka K. Complete removal of HIV-1 RNA and proviral DNA from semen reproduction technique using spermatozoa free from HIV-1. *AIDS*, 20: 967-973, 2006.

Marina S., Marina F., Alcolea R., Nadal J., Expósito R., Huguet J. Pregnancy following intracytoplasmic sperm injection from an HIV-1 seropositive man. *Human Reproduction,* 13 (11): 3247-3249, 1998.

Melo M.A.B, Mesenger M.,Bellver J., Remohi J., Pellicer A., Garrido N. Human immunodeficiency type-1 virus (HIV-1) infection in serodiscordant couples (SDCs) does not have an impact on embryo quality or intracytoplasmic sperm injection (ICSI) outcome. *Fertility and Sterility*, 89 (1): 141-150, 2008.

Morozumi K., Tateno H., Yanagida K., Katayose H., Kamiguchi Y., Sato A. Chromossomal analysis of mouse spermatozoa following physical and chemical treatments that are effective in inactivating HIV. *Zygote*, 12: 339-344, 2004.

Nahvi S., Flanigan T., Ca-Uvin S. Processing of semen from human immunodeficiency virus-seropositive men for use in insemination of seronegative women. *American Journal of Obstetrics and Gynecology*, 184 (3): 1048-1049, 2001.

Nakuda G.S., Pena J.E., Sauer M.V. Deaths of HIV-positive men in the context of assisted reproduction: five case studies from a single center. *AIDS patient care and DSTs*, 19 (11): 712-718, 2005.

Nicopoullos J.D.M., Frodsham L.C.G., Ramasay J.W.A., Almeida P.A., Rozis G., Gilling-Smith C. Synchronous sperm retrieval and sperm washing in an intracytoplasmic sperm injection cycle in an azoospermic man who was positive for human immunodeficiency virus. *Fertility and Sterility*, 81 (3): 670-674, 2004.

Peña J.E., Klein J., Thomton II M., Chang P.L., Sauer M.V. Successive pregnancies with delivery of two healthy infants in a couple who was discordant for human immunodeficiency virus infection. *Fertility and Sterility*, 78 (2): 421-423, 2002.

Peña J.E., Thornton M.H., Sauer M.V. Preliminary experience offering oocyte donation to human immunodeficiency virus-1 serodiscordant couples. A*rchieves of Gynecology and Obstetrics,* 268: 202-205, 2003.

Sauer M.V. Providing fertility care to those with HIV: time to re-examine healthycare policy. *The America Journal of Bioethics*, 3 (1): 33-40, 2003.

Semprini A.E and Levi-Setti P. Insemination of HIV-negative women with processed semen of HIV-positive partners. *Lancet,* 340 (8831): 1317-1319, 1992.

Terriou P., Auquier P., Chabert-Orsini V., Chinchole J.M., Cravello L., Giorgetti C., Halfon P., Salzmann J., Roulier R. Outcome of ICSI in HIV-1 infected women. *Human Reproduction,* 20 (10): 2838-2843, 2005.

Van Leeuwen E., Repping S., Prins J.M., Reiss P., van der Veen F. Assisted reproductive technologies to establish pregnancies in couples with an HIV-1-infected man. *The Journal of Netherlands Journal of Medicine,* 67(8): 322-327, 2009

UNAIDS/WHO. Status of the global HIV epidemic. Chapter 2, In: 2008 Report on the global AIDS epidemic. Accessed in November/06/2010, http://www.unaids.org/en/KnowledgeCentre/HIVData/GlobalReport/2008/2008_Global_report.asp.

In: In Vitro Fertilization
Editors: Samantha P. Steiger, pp. 109-122

ISBN 978-1-61209-961-3

Chapter VI

Proteomic Analysis of Embryos for Global Peptide Sequencing, Identification and Quantification of Multiple Proteins

Mukesh Kumar Gupta, Jin Woo Jung, Hoon Taek Lee and Kwang Pyo Kim*

Department of Molecular Biotechnology/Animal Biotechnology, Konkuk University, Hwayang-dong, Gwangjin-Gu, Seoul, South Korea

Abstract

Knowing what, where and when different proteins are expressed during embryonic development and how functional and structural alterations of proteins control the development programs are fundamental issues in developmental biology. Traditionally, this goal has been achieved by studying one or few proteins at a time, but a research tool that can handle several proteins in parallel would clearly be more valuable. Embryo proteomics is a rapidly emerging research field from the interface of proteomics and embryology that allows simultaneous identification and quantification of multiple proteins in embryonic samples. Besides, embryo proteomic data are essential for the completion of whole proteome catalog of any species because the expression of certain proteins are restricted to early embryonic developmental stages and are not expressed in somatic cells and tissues. Mass spectrometry (MS), applied as key techniques in proteomic research, is providing new insight into mechanism of developmental biology and is expected to improve the efficiency of assisted reproductive technologies (ART). Here, we provide some essential information about MS- based proteomics, and their applications to investigate embryo proteome. We also discuss the current limitations and measures that can increase our confidence in the accuracy of MS scans used in proteomic experiments.

* Correspondence: Kwang Pyo Kim (kimkp@konkuk.ac.kr) / Mukesh Kumar Gupta (goops@konkuk.ac.kr); Fax: +82-2-4578488; Tel: +82-2-4503694.

Introduction

The term "proteome" was first introduced in 1995 by Marc Wilkins to represent the "proteins expressed by a particular genome". It is now defined as the time- and cell-specific protein complement of the genome that encompass all proteins, including isoforms and post-translational modifications, that are expressed by the cell at a particular time point (Pandey and Mann, 2000). There are currently three widely accepted divisions of proteomics: 1) Clinical proteomics for investigating disease biomarkers; 2) Structural proteomics for analyzing and understanding the properties of cellular proteins; and 3) Functional proteomics for investigating the cell signaling mechanisms. A new research field, which may be called 'developmental proteomics' or 'embryo proteomics,' is now emerging from the interface between proteomics and developmental biology. It may be defined as the systematic analysis of cohorts of proteins expressed during development, aided by large-scale proteomic methods. In a broad sense, embryo proteomics can include all high-throughput approaches such as 2-dimensional gel electrophoresis (2DE), protein microarray, in silico proteomics and activity-based profiling.

Embryo proteomics is essential for the completion of a whole proteome catalog of any species because expressions of several proteins are restricted to early embryonic developmental stages and are not expressed in somatic cells and tissues (Gao et al., 2004; Ko, 2001). However, embryonic samples are rare materials that are difficult to obtain for ethical and technical reasons. The difficulty of obtaining early embryonic material is reflected in the current publicly available papers in which <1000 embryos were used to for whole proteomic analysis that could identify <50 proteins and mainly consisted of high abundant proteins. Application of matrix-assisted laser-desorption ionization time-of-flight (MALDI-TOF) approach of MS combined with 2DE for the separation of protein mixtures has enabled the identification and differential expression of 35 proteins during in vitro maturation of porcine oocytes (Ellederova et al., 2004), 24 proteins in porcine somatic nuclei exposed to oocyte extract system (Novak et al., 2004), 40 proteins during in vitro maturation of bovine oocytes (Bhojwani et al., 2006), 12 proteins in vitro maturation of mouse oocytes (Vitale et al., 2007) and 39 (Chae et al., 2006) to 43 (Lee et al., 2007c) proteins in extraembryonic tissue from cloned porcine embryos. More recently, surface-enhanced laser-desorption and ionization time-of-flight (SELDI-TOF) method has surfaced as a potential proteomic tool for biomarker discovery in limited amount of embryonic samples (Katz-Jaffe et al., 2005). This approach enabled the proteomic expression profiling of single human embryos (Katz-Jaffe et al., 2006a) and of soluble proteins secreted by the human and mouse embryos during in vitro culture (Katz-Jaffe et al., 2006b). However, SELDI-TOF produces only a pattern of peptides and small proteins that might be useful for discovering biomarkers of embryo quality but not for protein identification and quantification. Thus, although the use of SELDI-TOF in limited embryo samples is tantalizing, the reliability and reproducibility of data has been the subject of debate, given its limited sensitivity for low-abundance components and the limited robustness of the bioinformatics analysis (Baggerly et al., 2004; Combelles and Racowsky, 2006). We successfully applied 1DE followed by integrated liquid-chromatography-electrospray ionization-tendem MS (LC-ESI-MS/MS) for global peptide sequencing and quantification of embryonic proteins in porcine embryos. Through this approach we identified 1625 mammalian and 735 Sus scrofa proteins from porcine zygotes that included both cytosolic and membranous proteins (Gupta et al., 2009a). A similar approach was also applied in mouse oocyte that identified 2781 and 2973 proteins in germinal vesicle (GV) and Metaphase II (MII) stage oocytes, respectively (Wang et al., 2010). These reports are the highest reported number of proteins in one single experiment and thereby, demonstrated the potential and usefulness of embryo proteomics.

Application of Embryo Proteomics

The ultimate aim of proteomics is to create a complete three-dimensional map of the cells indicating proteins location, functions and interactions. High-throughput approaches of embryo proteomics can therefore, generate information about embryonic proteins and pathways that can give an integrated view of complex development processes. Indeed, the usefulness of proteomic approaches has been shown to understand the mechanism of embryonic development and identifying developmental deformities (Choi et al., 2008; Gupta et al., 2007; Chae et al., 2006; Chae et al., 2008; Cho et al., 2007; Chu et al., 2006; Katz-Jaffe et al., 2005; Lee et al., 2007c; Park et al., 2005; Park et al., 2004) in mammalian species. Even scientists using traditional model organisms, such as frog (Devreese et al., 2002), zebra fish (Tay et al., 2006), and Caenorhabditis elegans (Chu et al., 2006) have started to adopt proteomic approaches.

A thoroughly designed embryo proteomic experiment may decipher, 1) the functions of individual proteins, protein families as well as common proteins of one or more signaling pathways in the context of their activity in a particular development stage; 2) the role of post-translational modifications (PTMs) and protein interactions on the activity of developmentally important proteins, and 3) understanding the influence of transcriptional and translational regulation, RNA alternative splicing, compartmentalization, proteolysis, and the PTMs on the protein expression and their activity in the embryo. Nevertheless, the complexity of proteomes precludes addressing all these parameters in a single experiment and several approaches may be needed adopted to address each aspect of the proteome. For example, whole embryo can be subjected to proteomic analysis using a specific tool to either explore the expression level of several proteins or to identify the presence of a sequence isoforms in a given developmental stage under certain experimental condition or among different development stages. Moving beyond basic protein identification, investigations can also aim to describe all protein modifications and their changes in response to various experimental challenges to the embryos. Alternatively, cellular compartments of embryo can be isolated to build an inventory of their protein complement. If study on protein-protein interaction is desired, systematic purification of multi-protein complexes followed by the identification of their members would be required to build a protein-protein interaction map (Neubauer et al., 1998).

Available Tools for Embryo Proteomics

1. Gel Based Approaches

In earlier days and until relatively recently, profiling of protein expression in embryos and cells relied primarily on the use of two-dimensional polyacrylamide gel electrophoresis (2D PAGE) (Coenen et al., 2004). This approach involved solubilization of the entire protein contents of the cell population/ tissue/ embryos or biological fluid followed by their separation on 2D gels. The separated proteins are subsequently visualized using silver staining. However, this approach allows only a limited display of protein content that primarily consisted of relatively abundant proteins. An improvement of conventional 2D PAGE is the use of immobilized pH gradients (IPGs) in which the pH gradient is fixed within the acrylamide matrix (Chae et al., 2006; Lee et al., 2007b). However, the narrow dynamic range of 2-D gels again imposes limitations in separating the proteins with high or low molecular masses, extreme pIs (particularly basic proteins), high hydrophobic proteins, and the proteins of low abundance (Fountoulakis, 2001; Lubec et al., 2003). Consequently, this approach often tends to identify and frequently over-represent proteins that are more hydrophilic and relatively abundant. A further improvement in this approach is the use of so-called 'zoom gels' in which total protein content of the cell/embryo are first fractionated into narrow pH ranges under low resolution, and then each fraction is subjected to high-resolution separation by 2D PAGE (Zuo and Speicher, 2002). More recently, differential in-gel electrophoresis (DIGE) has emerged as a potential tool for differential protein expression analysis (Bhojwani et al., 2006). In this method, two or more pools of proteins are labeled with different fluorescent dyes, mixed and then separated in the same 2D gel. Differential expression of proteins is then aided by visual observation and fluorescent intensity of two fluorophore at same protein spot. However, even with all these improvements, 2D gels probably remain a rather low-throughput approach that requires a relatively large amount of sample. The latter is particularly important for embryo proteomics as embryo are generally procured in very limited amounts and it imposes a cost and time constraint.

2. MS-Based Approaches

MS analyses of proteins are carried out in the gas phase to measure the mass-to-charge ratio (m/z) of ionized peptides which is then utilized to obtain information about the proteins. The process involves: 1) protein sample preparation/fractionation by 1D SDS-PAGE or 2DE; 2) digestion of proteins to peptides using sequence specific protease such as trypsin, Lys-C, Asp-N or Glu-C endopeptidases; 3) peptide separation by high performance liquid chromatography (HPLC) or by ion exchange chromatography; 4) sample ionization by electrospray ionization (ESI) or matrix assisted laser desoprtion ionization (MALDI); 5) mass analysis by Quadrupole, or Time-of-Flight (TOF) or Ion trap or Fourier transform ion cyclotron (FT-MS) mass analyzers and; 6) bioinformatics based analysis of MS-generated data. The embryo sample can be prepared by extracting the total protein by standard method and, if necessary, can be stored in liquid nitrogen until use. The later is necessary because MS analysis generally require a large amount of embryos which are difficult to obtain in a single experiment. Once the desired amount of protein is collected, they can be pooled and subjected to 1D SDS-PAGE or 2DE depending on experimental design. The purpose of this step is to pre-fractionate the protein sample which aid protein identification by MS-analysis. Besides, 2DE allows intensity comparison of a protein spot in two different samples. Once the proteins in a protein spot are identified, one gets a fair estimation of differential protein expression of the identified protein. Of note, 1D SDS-PAGE does not give a good estimation of differential protein estimation because a particular band may contain several proteins all of which may not be differentially expressed. Following 1D SDS-PAGE or 2DE, the protein bands (in case of 1D SDS-PAGE) or spots of differential intensity (in case of 2DE) are cut out and proteins are digested individually with a protease enzyme to break them into smaller peptides. This is necessary primarily to prevent the clogging of the pipette and to maintain the desired flow of solution into the mass spectrometer for further analysis. To enable the clear reading, peptides must be purified at this stage by ion chromatography and may further be separated in second dimension by high performance liquid chromatography (HPLC) before injecting the sample into the mass spectrometer. The later is generally performed in LC-MS/MS method and therefore, HPLC machine is often integrated to the mass spectrometer.

Mass spectrometer consists of an ion source, a mass analyzer that measures the m/z ratio of the ionized sample, and a detector that registers the number of ions at each m/z value. Different types of mass spectrometers are available with different modalities for sample ionization and mass analysis and the choice of mass spectrometer depend on the experimental requirement. Currently, ESI and MALDI are most commonly used to volatize and ionize the peptides for mass spectrometric analysis. ESI ionizes the sample out of a solution and is therefore readily coupled to liquid-based (for example, chromatographic and electrophoretic) separation tools. On the other hand, MALDI sublimates and ionizes the samples out of a dry, crystalline matrix via laser pulses. Therefore, MALDI-MS is normally used to analyze relatively simple peptide mixtures that are difficult to ionize, whereas integrated liquid-chromatography ESI-MS systems (LC-MS) are preferred for the analysis of complex samples.

MALDI is usually coupled to TOF analyzers that measure the mass of intact peptides. The proteins are then identified by a method called peptide mapping, peptide-mass mapping or peptide-mass fingerprinting (PMF). In this method, molecular mass of each peptide, as determined by the MS, is matched with the calculated mass of each peptide listed in databases such as NCBI or EMBL to identify the protein. On the other hand, ESI is mostly coupled to ion traps or triple quadrupole instruments to generate fragment ion spectra [collision-induced (CID) spectra] of selected precursor ions. The proteins are then identified by matching the MS-generated CID spectra of peptides against comprehensive protein sequence databases using one of a number of different algorithms. Protein identification from ESI-MS/MS are generally more clear-cut than those achieved by mass mapping because, in addition to the peptide mass, the peak pattern in the CID spectrum also provides information about peptide sequence. Moreover, this can further be combined with multidimensional protein identification technology (MudPIT) to separate the peptide mixtures in two dimensions - first on the basis of their charge, and then on the basis of their hydrophobicity. In either method, peptide sequence information obtained from the -MS/MS experiment is converted into a full peptide sequence using bioinformatics tools to identify the proteins.

3. Non-Separation-Based Approaches

Direct protein profiling using MS or use of protein microarrays are other non-separation-based strategies in proteomics. Recently, it has been possible to in situ analyze the proteomics of tissues by imaging of protein expression using MS approach (Stoeckli et al., 2001). In this method, frozen tissue sections are applied on a MALDI plate and analyzed at regular spatial intervals. The mass spectra obtained at different intervals are then compared to obtain spatial distribution of individual masses across the tissue section. Mass profiles of tissue sections obtained from normal and abnormal tissues can then be compared to detect altered protein expression. Unfortunately, technical difficulties in processing the small sized embryos have so far limited its application in oocyte and embryos. Protein microarray is yet another important proteomic tool that can address many different features of proteins (Madoz-Gurpide et al., 2001) including their selective interactions with other biomolecules, such as other proteins, antibodies, or various small ligands. For assays of protein interaction, biochips that contain either peptides or proteins are being produced by several companies such as SomaLogic (http://www.somalogic.com/), Archemix (http://www.archemix.com/), Aspira Biosystems (http://www.aspirabio.com), and Phylos (http://www.phylos.com). One of the main challenges in protein biochips for global analysis of protein expression is the current lack of comprehensive sets of proteom-scale capturing agents such as antibodies. Inability of biochips to capture PTMs or specific protein isoforms further limits the use of protein microarrays. Consequently these techniques are still under experimental stage and have not yet been applied to embryos.

MS-Based Protein Profiling in Embryonic Samples

Protein profiling of oocytes and embryos can now be routinely characterized to some depth by methods described above. Coenen et al., (2004) had analyzed the protein profile of bovine oocytes using 2DE and found three major patterns of protein synthesis during the process of maturation. Ellederova et al., (2004) utilized both MALDI-TOF and LC-MS/MS for protein profiling of porcine oocyte during in vitro maturation of porcine oocyte and found that several proteins including peroxiredoxins, ubiquitin carboxyl-terminal hydrolase isozyme L1, and spermine synthase were even more abundant that actin protein. Massicott et al., (2006) also performed the protein profiling of bovine oocytes by 2DE combined with MALDI-TOF. The 2DE combined with LC-MS/MS has also been used for protein profiling of mouse oocytes (Vitale et al., 2007). Using reverse phase nanoLC-nanoESI-MS/MS LTQ ion-trap mass spectrometeric approach, we have recently created a proteome map of porcine embryos (Gupta et al., 2007; Jang et al., 2007a)and analyzed the protein profile of parthenogenetic and in vitro fertilized (IVF) embryos (Gupta et al., 2009a). This methodology required adoption of multiple strategies to increase the depth of the range and the total number of identified proteins. Firstly, given that porcine embryos contain ~ 273±16 ng of total proteins per embryo and limit of detection of LC-MS/MS falls in the range of 1-3 fmol (Giorgianni et al., 2004), proteins were extracted from a larger number of embryos (6000 per sample) so as to increase the probability of low abundant proteins getting detected. Second, presence of abundant proteins of zona pellucida on the surface of oocytes restricts the quantification of proteins (Ellederova et al., 2004). Furthermore, zona pellucida sperm-binding proteins are sulfated and heavily O-glycosylated proteins that causes spreading of proteins on the gel (Yurewicz et al., 1992). Therefore, we removed the zona-pellucida of embryos by a non-enzymatic method before subjecting them for protein extraction. Lastly, the total proteins that were obtained from zona-free embryos were separated by 1-DE into 16 fractions each of which were then individually digested by trypsin before being further separated by RP-LC. The separated tryptic digests were subsequently characterized by MS/MS. By this approach, we generated 54060 spectra, of which 4159 valid distinct peptides matched to NCBI database for mammalian proteins while 1346 valid distinct peptides matched to NCBI database for *S. scrofa* proteins. Analysis of these protein sequences against NCBI protein database lead to identification of 1083 mammalian proteins and 278 *S. scrofa* proteins with confidence level of >95%. The false positive rates were 4.14% for mammalian proteins and 2.66% for *S. scrofa* proteins, respectively. Among these proteins, 274 mammalian and 113 *S. scrofa* proteins had sequence coverage of >30% and included both cytoplasmic and nuclear proteins.

We also compared the proteome of parthenogentic and IVF embryos by quantifying the MS proteomics data by measuring peak heights and peptide counts (Jang et al., 2007b; Gupta et al., 2007). Both the coverage of unique peptides (that is, percentage of possible peptides per protein actually observed) and the total number of repeat observations of peptides was used for estimating the protein abundance. Furthermore, myoglobin and MAP3K synthetic peptides were used as internal standards to obtain qualitative information about peptide retention by reverse-phase chromatography, ionization efficiency, and fragmentation via collision-induced dissociation. Through this approach, we found that 924 mammalian and 221 *S. scrofa* proteins were differentially expressed between parthenogenetic and IVF embryos, using the cut-off filter of 2.0-fold or greater difference. Among these differentially expressed proteins, 474 mammalian and 97 *S. scrofa* proteins were up-regualted more than 10 folds while 62 mammalian and 9 *S. scrofa* proteins were down-regulated more than 10 folds in parthenogenetic embryos compared to IVF embryos. Functional annotation of differentially expressed proteins by bioinformatics tools revealed that proteins involved in cellular metabolism were mainly disrupted in parthenogenetic embryos and accounted for 47.5% of up-regulated proteins and 65.7% of down-regulated proteins. Proteins of signal transduction, embryonic development and metabolism of protein, RNA and DNA comprised 27.1% of up-regulated and 29.1% of down-regulated proteins. We found at least 26 proteins that are known to be related to pre-implantation development, placentation and post-implantation development. These proteins exert complex functions in signal-transduction pathways, and deranged protein levels may affect signal transduction and result in reduced embryonic development. Taken together, our data supported the proposal that mass spectrometry is a powerful tool for proteome analysis of porcine embryos to obtain vital new information for understanding the basic biology of embryonic development.

MS-Based Quantification and Differential Analysis of Protein Expression in Embryonic Samples

Simultaneous quantification of multiple proteins could be a very useful tool in cell signaling studies in embryos. Traditionally, this goal has been achieved by analyzing one or few proteins at a time or though quantification of mRNA transcripts by cDNA microarray or PCR-based approaches. While the former limits the number of proteins to be examined, interpretations from the later are based on the assumption that up- and down-regulation of mRNA accompanies functional changes in the cell which in fact, does not hold in all instances. Proteomics and proteomic techniques can provide information about several proteins at a time and therefore, are emerging as valuable tools for embryological research. In the most commonly used method for quantification and/or differential analysis of protein expression, the proteins in a sample are separated by 2DE, stained, and each observed protein spot is quantified by its staining intensity. Selected spots are then excised, digested and subjected to peptide-mass mapping by MALDI-TOF or peptide sequencing by ESI-MS/MS (Novak et al., 2004; Sutovsky et al., 2005). Using this approach, Ellederova et al., (2004) found that at least 13 proteins were differentially expressed between immature and matured porcine oocytes. However, in both MALDI- and ESI-MS, the relationship between the amount of analyte present and measured signal intensity is complex and therefore, signal intensity of a peptide ion does not directly indicate the absolute amount of protein present. Nonetheless, these strategies have been quite informative for differential expression analysis of proteins.

1. Absolute Quantification (AQUA)

Absolute quantification of one or more proteins by MS-based proteomics can be achieved by adding known amounts of isotopically labelled synthetic peptides (internal standards) into the peptide sample prior to its digestion and loading onto the column. The isotopically labeled internal standard mimic an expected proteolytic peptide but have a slightly different mass and therefore, produces a spectrum near to the peptide to be quantified. Since the concentration of internal standard is known, comparison of the two spectra would provide a measure of the endogenous peptide (Gerber et al., 2003). A method for large-scale absolute protein expression measurements (APEX) has also been described (Lu et al., 2007). Relying on the discriminating power of mass analyzers to select a specific analyte and on ion current measurements for quantification, the MS, in combination with appropriate stable isotope-labeled internal standards, also provides an alternative assay approach called selected reaction monitoring (SRM) or Multiple SRM (mSRM or MRM). This approach can be applied to the measurement of specific peptides in a complex mixtures such as trypic digest of cells and embryos (Anderson and Hunter, 2006). Hybrid methods have also been developed coupling MRM assays with enrichment of proteins by immunodepletion and size exclusion chromatography or enrichment of peptides by antibody capture (SISCAPA). We have recently shown the application of mSRM for porcine embryos for quantifying multiple cell signaling molecules (Gupta et al., 2008; Lee et al., 2007a).

One limitation of embryo proteomics is the difficulty in orthogonal verification of discovery findings by repeating LC-MS/MS experiment because it uses too much sample and immuno-based methods may not be possible due to lack of specific antibodies. We have recently shown that, in these circumstances, SRM is a viable approach - and perhaps the only option for the verification of LC-MS/MS shotgun discovery findings. At least in embryonic samples from porcine species, these measures were found to be useful in validating MS-identified differentially expressed proteins. Among the nine proteins analyzed by SRM assay, all the proteins that were found to be up- or down-regulated in MS experiment were also faithfully up- or down-regulated in SRM assay (Gupta et al., 2009b; Gupta et al., 2009a).

2. Relative Quantification

Relative quantification of proteins in an experimental group in relation to control group can be done by several approaches. One such approaches is stable-isotope dilution (Mirgorodskaya et al., 2000). In this method, after isolating the proteins, stable-isotope tags are introduced either enzymatically by transferring ^{18}O from water to peptides or chemically by using isotope-coded affinity tags or via metabolic labeling using heavy salts or amino acids. Since a mass spectrometer can differentiate the pairs of chemically identical analytes of different stable-isotope composition by their mass difference, the ratio of signal intensities for such analyte pairs accurately indicates the abundance ratio for the two analytes. Recently, another method called 'stable-isotope labelling with amino acids in cell culture', or SILAC, has also been described (Ong et al., 2002). This approach involves the addition of a stably labeled amino acid into the culture media. When cells are cultured in the cultured medium these labeled amino acids gets incorporated into the proteome of the cell. For analysis, the cell lysates from control and treatment groups are combined and MS-analysis is performed to compare the signal intensities and calculate the peptide ratio for each mass spectrum. Yet another method of relative quantification is ICAT ('isotope-coded affinity tag') that incorporates a label which is composed of three modular parts - an isotopically labelled linker between a biotin group and a thiol-specific (cysteine) reactant (Gygi et al., 1999). Two different isotopically labeled linkers are used to compare the peptides of two different protein populations, and the biotin group allows the selective capture and analysis of only the subset of peptides that contain the relatively rare cysteine residue. Although not been used in embryonic samples, theoretically these methods of relative quantifications are quite applicable to embryo culture systems.

MS-Based Analysis of PTMs in Embryonic Samples

Analysis of PTMs in embryonic samples is of particular importance in epigenetic studies (Das et al., 2010). Specific MS-based techniques have been developed that can scan the peptides for the presence of a particular PTM. Identification of PTMs is aided by computer-assisted interpretation using a variety of available algorithms. One strategy is that, instead of searching the database for non-modified peptides, the database search algorithms are instructed to also match the potentially modified peptides. A more functionally oriented strategy is to search for only one type of modification on all the proteins present in the sample. Such techniques are based usually on some form of affinity selection (e.g. modification specific antibody or chemical modification prior to MS) that is specific for the modification of interest and which is used to purify the 'sub-proteome' bearing this modification (Vitale et al., 2007). More recently, protein microarrays have also been used to simultaneously analyze the PTM of histone proteins. The MODified Histone Peptide Array^{TM}, marketed by ActiveMotif (www.activemotif.com), can be used to screen antibodies, proteins and enzymes for interactions with hisones and their PTMs. Each array contains 384 different histone modification combinations for acetylation, methylation, phosphorylation and citrullination modifications on the N-terminal tails of histones H2A, H2B, H3 and H4. the array contains up to four modifications per 19 mer peptide to allow the study of not only individual sites but also the effects of neighboring modifications on recognition and binding. Importantly, the array protocol works like a Western blot and either ECL-based or colorimetric detection system can be used and no special equipment is needed.

Limitations and Pitfalls of Embryo Proteomics

Proteomic science is relatively new to developmental biology and the development of sensitive techniques and methods for protein quantification and identification are still under way. A major problem with utilization of large scale proteomic tool to embryos is the limited availability of samples for analysis and limited sensitivity of the MS. Currently MS can identify 1-10 fmol of a peptide loaded on a chromatography column in routine analysis. Analysis of a protein that is present at a level of 1000 copies per cell would theoretically require 10^6 cells to start with, assuming no losses during protein purification. In embryonic system a minimum of 500-1500 oocytes or more are required to obtain reliable data. The depth and range of identified proteins from embryonic samples can be increased by removing highly abundant protein such as zona pellucida using a non-enzymatic method. Another limitation of mass spectrometry is that the sequence databases that are used to identify proteins are still far from optimal for proteomics experiments and this severely hinders the proteomic study in farm animals. In the quest to characterize the proteome of given embryo, it should also be remembered that the proteome is dynamic and will immediately reflect the environment in which it is studied. In response to internal or external signals, a protein can be modified by PTMs, undergo translocations within the cell, and also be synthesized or degraded at various stages of embryo development. Considering all the possibilities, it is likely that any genome can potentially give rise to a very large number of proteomes which might be hard to interpret.

Conclusion

MS-based proteomics can yield very detailed information about a protein sample, including an extensive analysis of protein modifications that can provide vital information on developmental process. However, several limitations exist and one need to be careful as to what can be concluded from a protein analysis. With the rapid growth in the embryo proteomics, it can be expected that proteomic studies will soon replace and/or aid genomic study to substantially increase our understanding of complex biological processes of embryonic development.

References

Anderson, L., and Hunter, C.L. (2006) Quantitative mass spectrometric multiple reaction monitoring assays for major plasma proteins. *Mol Cell Proteomics* 5:573-588.

Baggerly, K.A., Morris, J.S., and Coombes, K.R. (2004) Reproducibility of SELDI-TOF protein patterns in serum: comparing datasets from different experiments. *Bioinformatics* 20:777-785.

Bhojwani, M., Rudolph, E., Kanitz, W., Zuehlke, H., Schneider, F., and Tomek, W. (2006) Molecular analysis of maturation processes by protein and phosphoprotein profiling during in vitro maturation of bovine oocytes: a proteomic approach. *Cloning Stem Cells* 8:259-274.

Chae, J.I., Cho, S.K., Seo, J.W., Yoon, T.S., Lee, K.S., Kim, J.H., Lee, K.K., Han, Y.M., and Yu, K. (2006) Proteomic analysis of the extraembryonic tissue from cloned porcine embryos. *Mol Cell Proteomics* 5:1559-1566.

Chae, J.I., Cho, Y.K., Cho, S.K., Kim, J.H., Han, Y.M., Koo, D.B., and Lee, K.K. (2008) Proteomic analysis of pancreas derived from adult cloned pig. *Biochem Biophys Res Commun* 366:379-387.

Cho, S.K., Kim, J.H., Park, J.Y., Choi, Y.J., Bang, J.I., Hwang, K.C., Cho, E.J., Sohn, S.H., Uhm, S.J., Koo, D.B., Lee, K.K., Kim, T., and Kim, J.H. (2007) Serial cloning of pigs by somatic cell nuclear transfer: restoration of phenotypic normality during serial cloning. *Dev Dyn* 236:3369-3382.

Choi, Y.J., Uhm, S.J., Song, S.J., Song, H., Park, J.K., Kim, T., Park, C., and Kim, J.H. (2008) Cytochrome c upregulation during capacitation and spontaneous acrosome reaction determines the fate of pig sperm cells: linking proteome analysis. *J Reprod Dev* 54:68-83.

Chu, D.S., Liu, H., Nix, P., Wu, T.F., Ralston, E.J., Yates, J.R., 3rd, and Meyer, B.J. (2006) Sperm chromatin proteomics identifies evolutionarily conserved fertility factors. *Nature* 443:101-105.

Coenen, K., Massicotte, L., and Sirard, M.A. (2004) Study of newly synthesized proteins during bovine oocyte maturation in vitro using image analysis of two-dimensional gel electrophoresis. *Mol Reprod Dev* 67:313-322.

Combelles, C.M., and Racowsky, C. (2006) Protein expression profiles of early embryos--an important step in the right direction: just not quite ready for prime time. *Fertil Steril* 86:493; author reply 493.

Das, Z.C., Gupta, M.K., Uhm, S.J., and Lee, H.T. (2010) Increasing histone acetylation of cloned embryos, but not donor cells, by sodium butyrate improves their in vitro development in pigs. *Cell Reprogram* 12:95-104.

Devreese, B., Janssen, K.P., Vanrobaeys, F., Van Herp, F., Martens, G.J., and Van Beeumen, J. (2002) Automated nanoflow liquid chromatography-tandem mass spectrometry for a differential display proteomic study on Xenopus laevis neuroendocrine cells. *J Chromatogr A* 976:113-121.

Ellederova, Z., Halada, P., Man, P., Kubelka, M., Motlik, J., and Kovarova, H. (2004) Protein patterns of pig oocytes during in vitro maturation. *Biol Reprod* 71:1533-1539.

Fountoulakis, M. (2001) Proteomics: current technologies and applications in neurological disorders and toxicology. *Amino Acids* 21:363-381.

Gao, L., Sun, C., Qiu, H.L., Liu, H., Shao, H.J., Wang, J., and Li, W.X. (2004) Cloning and characterization of a novel human zinc finger gene, hKid3, from a C2H2-ZNF enriched human embryonic cDNA library. *Biochem Biophys Res Commun* 325:1145-1152.

Gerber, S.A., Rush, J., Stemman, O., Kirschner, M.W., and Gygi, S.P. (2003) Absolute quantification of proteins and phosphoproteins from cell lysates by tandem MS. *Proc Natl Acad Sci U S A* 100:6940-6945.

Giorgianni, F., Cappiello, A., Beranova-Giorgianni, S., Palma, P., Trufelli, H., and Desiderio, D.M. (2004) LC-MS/MS analysis of peptides with methanol as organic modifier: improved limits of detection. *Anal Chem* 76:7028-7038.

Gupta, M.K., Jang, J.M., Jung, J.W., Uhm, S.J., Kim, K.P., and Lee, H.T. (2008) Simultaneous quantification of multiple proteins in porcine parthenotes by multiple selected reaction monitoring. *Reprod Fertil Dev* 20:166.

Gupta, M.K., Jang, J.M., Jung, J.W., Uhm, S.J., Kim, K.P., and Lee, H.T. (2009a) Proteomic analysis of parthenogenetic and in vitro fertilized porcine embryos. *Proteomics* 9:2846-2860.

Gupta, M.K., Jung, J.W., Uhm, S.J., Kim, K.P., and Lee, H.T. (2007) Embryo Proteomics: What it has got to offer? *Proceedings of the international symposium of research center for transgenic cloned pigs*:49.

Gupta, M.K., Jung, J.W., Uhm, S.J., Lee, H., Lee, H.T., and Kim, K.P. (2009b) Combining selected reaction monitoring with discovery proteomics in limited biological samples. *Proteomics* 9:4834-4836.

Gygi, S.P., Rist, B., Gerber, S.A., Turecek, F., Gelb, M.H., and Aebersold, R. (1999) Quantitative analysis of complex protein mixtures using isotope-coded affinity tags. *Nat Biotechnol* 17:994-999.

Jang, J.M., Gupta, M.K., Jung, J.W., Uhm, S.J., Kim, K.P., and Lee, H.T. (2007a) Global peptide sequencing and quantification of proteins in porcine parthenotes by proteomics. *Reprod Fertil Dev* 19:119.

Jang, J.M., Gupta, M.K., Jung, J.W., Uhm, S.J., Kim, K.P., and Lee, H.T. (2007b) Multiple Selected Reaction Monitoring of cell signaling molecules in porcine embryos. *Proceedings of the KU-UW symposium:35*.

Katz-Jaffe, M.G., Gardner, D.K., and Schoolcraft, W.B. (2006a) Proteomic analysis of individual human embryos to identify novel biomarkers of development and viability. *Fertil Steril* 85:101-107.

Katz-Jaffe, M.G., Linck, D.W., Schoolcraft, W.B., and Gardner, D.K. (2005) A proteomic analysis of mammalian preimplantation embryonic development. *Reproduction* 130:899-905.

Katz-Jaffe, M.G., Schoolcraft, W.B., and Gardner, D.K. (2006b) Analysis of protein expression (secretome) by human and mouse preimplantation embryos. *Fertil Steril* 86:678-685.

Ko, M.S. (2001) Embryogenomics: developmental biology meets genomics. *Trends Biotechnol* 19:511-518.

Lee, H.T., Jang, J.M., Jung, J.W., Uhm, S.J., Kim, K.P., and Gupta, M.K. (2007a) Multiple Selected Reaction Monitoring: as a tool for quantification of proteins in Porcine Embryos. Proceedings of the 4th annual meeting of the Asian Reproductive *Biotechnology Society*:5.

Lee, S.J., Kim, K.H., Park, J.S., Jung, J.W., Kim, Y.H., Kim, S.K., Kim, W.S., Goh, H.G., Kim, S.H., Yoo, J.S., Kim, D.W., and Kim, K.P. (2007b) Comparative analysis of cell surface proteins in chronic and acute leukemia cell lines. *Biochem Biophys Res Commun* 357:620-626.

Lee, S.Y., Park, J.Y., Choi, Y.J., Cho, S.K., Ahn, J.D., Kwon, D.N., Hwang, K.C., Kang, S.J., Paik, S.S., Seo, H.G., Lee, H.T., and Kim, J.H. (2007c) Comparative proteomic analysis associated with term placental insufficiency in cloned pig. *Proteomics* 7:1303-1315.

Lu, P., Vogel, C., Wang, R., Yao, X., and Marcotte, E.M. (2007) Absolute protein expression profiling estimates the relative contributions of transcriptional and translational regulation. *Nat Biotechnol* 25:117-124.

Lubec, G., Krapfenbauer, K., and Fountoulakis, M. (2003) Proteomics in brain research: potentials and limitations. *Prog Neurobiol* 69:193-211.

Madoz-Gurpide, J., Wang, H., Misek, D.E., Brichory, F., and Hanash, S.M. (2001) Protein based microarrays: a tool for probing the proteome of cancer cells and tissues. *Proteomics* 1:1279-1287.

Massicotte, L., Coenen, K., Mourot, M., and Sirard, M.A. (2006) Maternal housekeeping proteins translated during bovine oocyte maturation and early embryo development. *Proteomics* 6:3811-3820.

Mirgorodskaya, O.A., Kozmin, Y.P., Titov, M.I., Korner, R., Sonksen, C.P., and Roepstorff, P. (2000) Quantitation of peptides and proteins by matrix-assisted laser desorption/ionization mass spectrometry using (18)O-labeled internal standards. *Rapid Commun Mass Spectrom* 14:1226-1232.

Neubauer, G., King, A., Rappsilber, J., Calvio, C., Watson, M., Ajuh, P., Sleeman, J., Lamond, A., and Mann, M. (1998) Mass spectrometry and EST-database searching allows characterization of the multi-protein spliceosome complex. *Nat Genet* 20:46-50.

Novak, S., Paradis, F., Savard, C., Tremblay, K., and Sirard, M.A. (2004) Identification of porcine oocyte proteins that are associated with somatic cell nuclei after co-incubation. *Biol Reprod* 71:1279-1289.

Ong, S.E., Blagoev, B., Kratchmarova, I., Kristensen, D.B., Steen, H., Pandey, A., and Mann, M. (2002) Stable isotope labeling by amino acids in cell culture, SILAC, as a simple and accurate approach to expression proteomics. *Mol Cell Proteomics* 1:376-386.

Pandey, A., and Mann, M. (2000) Proteomics to study genes and genomes. *Nature* 405:837-846.

Park, M.R., Cho, S.K., Lee, S.Y., Choi, Y.J., Park, J.Y., Kwon, D.N., Son, W.J., Paik, S.S., Kim, T., Han, Y.M., and Kim, J.H. (2005) A rare and often unrecognized cerebromeningitis and hemodynamic disorder: a major cause of sudden death in somatic cell cloned piglets. *Proteomics* 5:1928-1939.

Park, M.R., Cho, S.K., Park, J.Y., Lee, S.Y., Choi, Y.J., Kwon, D.N., Son, W.J., Seo, H.G., and Kim, J.H. (2004) Detection of rare Leydig cell hypoplasia in somatic cell cloned male piglets. *Zygote* 12:305-313.

Stoeckli, M., Chaurand, P., Hallahan, D.E., and Caprioli, R.M. (2001) Imaging mass spectrometry: a new technology for the analysis of protein expression in mammalian tissues. *Nat Med* 7:493-496.

Sutovsky, P., Manandhar, G., Laurincik, J., Letko, J., Caamano, J.N., Day, B.N., Lai, L., Prather, R.S., Sharpe-Timms, K.L., Zimmer, R., and Sutovsky, M. (2005) Expression and proteasomal degradation of the major vault protein (MVP) in mammalian oocytes and zygotes. *Reproduction* 129:269-282.

Tay, T.L., Lin, Q., Seow, T.K., Tan, K.H., Hew, C.L., and Gong, Z. (2006) Proteomic analysis of protein profiles during early development of the zebrafish, Danio rerio. *Proteomics* 6:3176-3188.

Vitale, A.M., Calvert, M.E., Mallavarapu, M., Yurttas, P., Perlin, J., Herr, J., and Coonrod, S. (2007) Proteomic profiling of murine oocyte maturation. *Mol Reprod Dev* 74:608-616.

Wang, S., Kou, Z., Jing, Z., Zhang, Y., Guo, X., Dong, M., Wilmut, I., and Gao, S. (2010) Proteome of mouse oocytes at different developmental stages. *Proc Natl Acad Sci U S A* 107:17639-17644.

Yurewicz, E.C., Pack, B.A., and Sacco, A.G. (1992) Porcine oocyte zona pellucida M(r) 55,000 glycoproteins: identification of O-glycosylated domains. *Mol Reprod Dev* 33:182-188.

Zuo, X., and Speicher, D.W. (2002) Comprehensive analysis of complex proteomes using microscale solution isoelectrofocusing prior to narrow pH range two-dimensional electrophoresis. *Proteomics* 2:58-68.

In: In Vitro Fertilization
Editor: Samantha P. Steiger, pp. 123-129
ISBN 978-1-61209-961-3

Chapter VII

The Impact of Laparoscopic Ovarian Cystectomy for Infertile Woman with Endometriomas Prior to IVF/ICSI Cycles

Chin-Jung Wang and Hsing-Tse Yu
Department of Obstetrics and Gynecology, Chang Gung Memorial Hospital at Linkou and Chang Gung University College of Medicine, Taoyuan, Taiwan

Abstract

Endometriosis is a common, benign, chronic gynecological disorder frequently associated with dysmenorrhea, pelvic pain, and infertility. The prevalence of endometriosis approaches 10–15% of all women of reproductive age while it has been reported that 25–40%of women within fertility have endometriosis. Current guidelines for the treatment of endometriosis include medical or surgical therapies. However, medical treatment has a limited role in the treatment of endometriosis that only offers symptomatic control. Associated with many advantages over traditional abdominal methods, including less hospitalization, smaller incisions, faster recovery time, and faster return to work, the laparoscopic approach for endometriosis has been now widely accepted. Therefore, laparoscopic surgery has traditionally been the standard treatment for patients with endometriosis. Until now, there is no consensus regarding the influence of previous surgery for endometriomas on ovarian function. Some investigators suggested that in vitro fertilization (IVF) outcome is compromised by previous ovarian surgery. Conversely, no adverse impact of prior surgery for endometriosis on ovarian reserve and response to controlled ovarian hyperstimulation (COH) has also been reported. The role of operative laparoscopy before or after IVF in women accompanied with ovarian endometrioma is more complicated. The recent guideline for management of endometriosis in women requiring IVF recommend surgery only carried out in the presence of large ovarian endometrioma. Hence, it needs thorough evaluation in managing ovarian endometriomas for infertile women.

Introduction

Endometriosis is a common, benign, chronic gynecological disorder frequently associated with dysmenorrheal and infertility. Endometriosis is defined as the presence of endometrial glandular and stromal cells outside their normal location of uterus, which include the ovaries, peritoneum. The pathogenesis of endometriosis is poorly understood; however, there is an inflammatory process for ectopic endometrial fragments to adhere, invade, and develop that results in dense adhesion between normal ovarian tissue and endometrioma. Therefore, there might be inadvertent removal of a consistent amount of normal ovarian tissue during cystectomy, potentially causing a reduction of ovarian function.

At present, the prevalence of endometriosis approaches 10–15% of all women of reproductive age [1] while it has been reported that one-third of women with endometriosis have ovarian endometriomas [2]. Current guidelines for the treatment of endometriosis include medical or surgical therapies. However, medical treatment has a limited role in the treatment of endometriosis that only offers symptomatic control. Surgical intervention has been demonstrated to be an effective treatment for ovarian endometriomas. Associated with many advantages over traditional abdominal methods, including less hospitalization, smaller incisions, faster recovery time, and faster return to work, the laparoscopic approach for endometriosis has been now widely accepted. Nevertheless, some investigations have suggested that laparoscopic surgery before IVF/ICSI might cause a reduction of ovarian function and impair ovarian responsiveness to hyperstimulation [3,4]. Until, now, there is no consensus regarding the guideline for the management of ovarian endometriomas prior to IVF/ICSI. Factors affecting the choice of decision making include patients' age, baseline ovarian reserve, history of previous ovarian surgery, the response for hyperstimulation in previous IVF/ICSI , and the size of ovarian endometriomas. In this regard, we will investigate whether laparoscopic cystectomy for ovarian endometriomas is needed for the infertile women prior to IVF/ICSI cycles and focus on the impact of previous laparoscopic surgery for IVF/ICSI outcomes.

Pathogenesis of Endometriosis-Related Subfertility

Many studies demonstrated that women with endometriosis have a lower fecundity than normal group, but the cause–effect relationship between endometriosis and infertility is controversial. Saito et al found that oxidative stress markers such as 8-hydroxy-2-nonenal, and 4-hydroxy-2-nonenal were significantly elevated in granulose cells of patients with endometriosis [5]. Gupta also noted that elevated reactive oxygen species causing oxidative stress are produced from endometrioma cells [6]. Oxidative stress play a large role in endometriosis-associated infertility owing to inducing oocyte degeneration and apoptosis through disturbing the meiotic spindle. In addition, reactive oxygen species might lead to cell death by increased membrane permeability, degraded membrane integrity, inactivated enzymes and structural damage of the DNA. Severe oxidative stress can have negative impact on the acrosome reaction and sperm–oocyte fusion. Consequently, it interferes with IVF by reduced fertilization rate, increased embryo fragmentation, and poor quality embryos.

Besides, endometriosis is associated with an inflammatory change in the follicular fluid and peritoneal fluid. It has been shown that several various components of immunity such as interleukins IL-6, IL-1b, IL-10, and tumor necrosis factor-a (TNF-a) are elevated in the follicular fluid with endometriosis patients during IVF/ICSI [7-9]. These cytokines may be responsible for alternations of the granulose cell cycles leading to fertility and fertilizing capacity. Moreover, elevated levels of TNF-a in the peritoneal fluid resulting in adverse effects on sperm function and integrity ,and other cytokines, such IL-1 and IL-6 in negative effects on sperm motility in the uterus might be thought to contribute to the subfertility of endometriosis patients [10,11].

Management of Ovarian Endometriomas Prior to IVF/ICSI

The treatment of ovarian endometrioms prior to IVF/ICSI is still controversial. The management of ovarian endometriomas prior to IVF/ICSI includes medical treatment or surgery. Medical treatment only offers profits for prevention of recurrence of endometriosis and the reduction of tumor size. Most ovarian endometriomas has poor response to medical treatment. Thus, medical treatment should not be considered as the standard treatment in infertile women. After a number of studies pointed that there are some benefits in the number of embryos transferred, pregnancy rate, and clinical pregnancy rate in the women who underwent surgical treatment of endometrioma comparing the non-treated endometrioma, surgery is adopted in the management of endometrioma before starting IVF/ICSI [4, 12-14].

Wong and coworkers described that the overall pregnancy rate was significantly higher in patients younger than 39 years of age who underwent conservative laparoscopy for ovarian endometriomas comparing with patients who had present ovarian endometriomas during ovarian hyperstimulation(65% vs 39%; P = .05) (4). They conducted that removal of endometriomas might be beneficial for pregnancy outcome prior to IVF/ICSI, however, this study was a retrospective cohort study. In contrast, some studies demonstrated that laparoscopic cystectomy had detrimental effect on ovarian response in the following IVF/ICSI cycles [3,15].

Suganuma et al indicated that women who underwent surgery for ovarian endometrial cysts were found to have significantly fewer retrieved follicles compared with patients who did not undergo pretreatment and confirmed ovarian endometriosis at oocyte retrieval in a retrospective case-controlled study. According to the recently published systemic reviewed article [16], only one randomized controlled trial has been conducted comparing conservative laparoscopy for the patients with ovarian endometriomas of which size was between 3cm and 6cm before commencing IVF/ICSI [17]. They noted no difference in fertilization, pregnancy and implantation rates between two groups, however, ovarian surgery resulted in longer stimulation, higher FSH requirement and lower oocyte number. Therefore, the European Society of Human Reproduction and Embryology (ESHRE) guidelines recommend laparoscopic ovarian cystectomy if the endometrioma is $\geq$4 cm in diameter in order to confirm the diagnosis histologically, to reduce the risk of infection, to improve access to follicles and possibly to improve ovarian response.

Operative Technique of Laparoscopic Cystectomy in Endometriosis

The procedures for the treatment of ovarian endometriomas include either excision of the cyst capsule or drainage and electrocoagulation of the cyst wall. The disadvantage of excision technique is to inadvertently remove a consistent amount of normal ovarian tissue during cystectomy. Ablative techniques have the potential disadvantages of extensive thermal effect causing the damage of normal ovarian tissue. According to the recently published systemic reviewed article, Hart RJ et al conducted that excision surgery for ovarian endometriomas provides for a more favorable outcome than drainage and ablation with regard to the recurrence of the endometrioma, recurrence of pain symptoms, and in women who were previously subfertile, subsequent spontaneous pregnancy [18].

The surgical technique of ovarian cyst excision by laparoscopy is usually using a stripping technique [19, 20]. In brief, laparoscopic examination of the pelvis and lower abdomen is performed to determine the accessibility of the surgical field. Three or four trocars are used according to complexity of pelvis. A disposable laparoscopic grasper, scissors, and suction-irrigator are used to perform various procedures such as holding, cutting, exploring and dissecting. A sharp cortical incision is made by unipolar scissors and a cleavage plane is identified. The capsule of the endometrioma is then enucleated and stripped from the normal ovarian tissue. Large bleeders are coagulated using bipolar forceps with an electrosurgical bipolar unit (Elmed, Addison, IL). Complete hemostasis and approximation of ovarian defect are achieved using a 3–0 monofilament poliglecaprone 25 suture (Monocryl; Ethicon Inc., Somerville, NJ, USA) on a large curved needle following the principles of laparotomy. The specimens are removed from the abdomen using a disposable endobag for the purpose of avoiding contaminating the abdominal wall.

The possible drawback of the laparoscopic stripping technique might be associated with loss of follicles and damage to the ovarian stroma [21]. The average time for ovarian function recovery is two menstrual cycles. Candiani et al. reported that reduced ovulation and ovarian volume came about over time after the second postoperative menstruation [22]. Exacoustos et al. reported a similar finding that a significant reduction in ovarian volume was noted after laparoscopic endometrioma removal by stripping [23]. However, some patients have severe ovarian damage following surgery for endometriomas. The incidence of severe ovarian damage after surgeries was estimated to be appproximately 13% by Benaglia et al[24]. In ninety-three women who underwent surgery for endometriomas, twelve patients had absence of follicular growth in operated ovaries even three years after ovarian surgery. Therefore, physicians should be aware that laparoscopic conservative surgery for endometriosis is a challenging task.

The Impact of Previous Conservative Surgery for Endometriosis on IVF-ICSI Outcome

The issue of previous conservative surgery for endometriosis on IVF/ICSI outcome is of a debate. For example, Loo et al. showed the reduced available oocytes and embryos accompanied with lower fertilization and implantation rate compared with tubal control group [25]. Ragni et al. reported that laparoscopic enucleation of ovarian endometrioma reduced the ovarian response to COH [26]. Nevertheless, these studies conducted that the high-quality embryos and the chance of pregnancy were not affected. On the other hand, several studies also reported that the number of oocytes and embryos were not decreased in infertile women committed to IVF–ET treatment after laparoscopic cystectomy [27, 28]. Bilateral lesions account for 19–28% in patients with ovarian endometriosis [29]. The severity of ovarian lesions (bilateral vs. unilateral) is theoretically an important factor for ovarian reserve after conservative surgery. Esinler et al. reported that laparoscopic endometrioma cystectomy diminished ovarian reserve in patients who underwent bilateral cystectomy compared with a unilateral group. Nevertheless, the pregnancy outcome was not affected bythe diminished ovarian reserve [30].

Medical Treatment after Laparoscopic Cystectomy for Endometriomas Following IVF/ICSI Program

Pre-treatment and post-operative hypoestrogenic agent administration for endometriosis is frequently combined with laparoscopic procedures, especial in advanced endometriosis. Vercellini et al reviewed that the overall pregnancy rate was 18.1% in the patients with post-operative medical treatment and 22.9% in the patients underwent conservative surgery only [2]. Another study also showed that there was not enough available evidence to support that hypoestrogenic agent combined with surgery for endometriosis provided significant clinical advantages [31].

References

[1] Moen MH. Is a long period without childbirth a risk factor for developing endometriosis? *Hum. Reprod.* 1991;6:1404–7.

[2] Vercellini P, Chapron C, De Giorgi O, Consonni D, Frontino G, Crosignani PG. Coagulation or excision of ovarian endometriomas? *Am. J. Obstet. Gynecol.* 2003;188:606–10.

[3] Ho HY, Lee RK, Hwu YM, Lin MH, Su JT, Tsai YC. Poor response of ovaries with endometrioma previously treated with cystectomy to controlled ovarian hyperstimulation. *J. Assist. Reprod. Genet.* 2002;19:507–11.

[4] Wong BC, Gillman NC, Oehninger S, Gibbons WE, Stadtmauer LA. Results of in vitro fertilization in patients with endometriomas: is surgical removal bene- ficial? *Am. J. Obstet. Gynecol.* 2004;191:597–606.

[5] Saito H, Seino T, Kaneko T, Nakahara K, Toya M, Kurachi H. Endometriosis and oocyte quality. *Gynecol. Obstet. Invest.* 2002;53(Suppl 1):46–51.

[6] Gupta S, Agarwal A, Krajcir N, Alvarez JG. Role of oxidative stress in endometriosis. *Reprod .Biomed. Online* 2006;13:126–34.

[7] Bedaiwy MA, Falcone T, Sharma RK, Goldberg JM, Attaran M, Nelson DR, et al. Prediction of endometriosis with serum and peritoneal fluidmarkers: a prospective controlled trial. *Hum. Reprod.* 2002;17:426–31.
[8] Pellicer A, Albert C, Mercader A, Bonilla-Musoles F, Remohi J, Simon C. The follicular and endocrine environment in women with endometriosis: local and systemic cytokine production. *Fertil. Steril.* 1998;70:425–31.
[9] Punnonen J, Teisala K, Ranta H, Bennett B, Punnonen R. Increased levels of interleukin-6 and interleukin-10 in the peritoneal fluid of patients with endometriosis. *Am. J. Obstet. Gynecol.* 1996;174:1522–6.
[10] Reeve L, Lashen H, Pacey AA. Endometriosis affects sperm-endosalpingeal interactions. *Hum. Reprod.* 2005;20:448–51.
[11] Yoshida S, Harada T, Iwabe T, Taniguchi F, Mitsunari M, Yamauchi N,et al. A combination of interleukin-6 and its soluble receptor impairs sperm motility: implications in infertility associated with endometriosis. *Hum. Reprod.* 2004;19:1821–5.
[12] Tinkanen H, Kujansuu E. In vitro fertilization in patients with ovarian endometriomas. *Acta Obstet. Gynecol. Scand.* 2000;79:119–22.
[13] Garcia-Velasco JA, Mahutte NG, Corona J, Zuniga V, Giles J, Arici A, et al. Removal of endometriomas before in vitro fertilization does not improve fertility outcomes: a matched, case-control study. *Fertil. Steril.* 2004;81:1194–7.
[14] Pabuccu R, Onalan G, Goktolga U, Kucuk T, Orhon E, Ceyhan T. Aspiration of ovarian endometriomas before intracytoplasmic sperm injection. *Fertil. Steril.* 2004;82:705–11.
[15] Suganuma N, Wakahara Y, Ishida D, Asano M, Kitagawa T, Katsumata Y, et al. Pretreatment for ovarian endometrial cyst before in vitro fertilization. *Gynecol. Obstet. Invest.* 2002;54(Suppl. 1):36–42.
[16] Tsoumpou I, Kyrgiou M, Gelbaya TA, Nardo LG. The effect of surgical treatment for endometrioma on in vitro fertilization outcomes: a systematic review and meta-analysis. *Fertil. Steril.* 2009;92(1):75-87
[17] Demirol, A., Guven, S., Baykal, C., Gurgan, T. Effect of endometrioma cystectomy on IVF outcome: a prospective randomized study. *Reprod. Biomed. Online* 2005;12, 639–643.
[18] Hart RJ, Hickey M, Maouris P, Buckett W. Excisional surgery versus ablative surgery for ovarian endometriomata. Cochrane Database Syst Rev. 2008 Apr 16;(2):CD004992.
[19] Nezhat C, Crowgey SR, Nezhat F. Videolaparoscopy for the treatment of endometriosis associated with infertility. *Fertil. Steril.* 1989;51:237–40.
[20] Martin DC. Laparoscopic treatment of ovarian endometriomas. *Clin. Obstet. Gynecol.* 1991;34:452–9.
[21] Hachisuga T, Kawarabayashi T. Histopathological analysis of laparoscopically treated ovarian endometriotic cysts with special reference to loss of follicles. *Hum. Reprod.* 2002;17:432–5.
[22] Candiani M, Barbieri M, Bottani B, Bertulessi C, Vignali M, Agnoli B, et al. Ovarian recovery after laparoscopic enucleation of ovarian cysts: insights from echographic short-term postsurgical follow-up. *J. Minim. Invasive Gynecol.* 2005;12:409–14.
[23] Exacoustos C, Zupi E, Amadio A, Szabolcs B, De Vivo B, Marconi D, et al. Laparoscopic removal of endometriomas: sonographic evaluation of residual functioning ovarian tissue. *Am. J. Obstet. Gynecol.* 2004;191:68–72.

[24] Benaglia L, Somigliana E, Vighi V, Ragni G, Vercellini P, Fedele L.Rate of severe ovarian damage following surgery for endometriomas. *Hum. Reprod.* 2010 Mar;25(3):678-82.

[25] Loo TC, Lin MY, Chen SH, Chung MT, Tang HH, Lin LY, Tsai YC. Endometrioma undergoing laparoscopic ovarian cystectomy: its influence on the outcome of in vitro fertilization and embryo transfer (IVF-ET). *J. Assist. Reprod. Genet.* 2005 ;22(9-10):329-33.

[26] Ragni G, Somigliana E, Benedetti F, Paffoni A, Vegetti W, Restelli L, et al. Damage to ovarian reserve associated with laparoscopic excision of endometriomas: a quantitative rather than a qualitative injury. *Am. J. Obstet. Gynecol.* 2005;193:1908–14

[27] Canis M, Pouly JL, Tamburro S, Mage G, Wattiez A, Bruhat MA: Ovarian response during IVF-embryo transfer cycles after laparoscopic ovarian cystectomy for endometriotic cysts of >3 cm in diameter. *Hum. Reprod.* 2001;16:2583–2586

[28] Marconi G, Vilela M, Quintana R, Sueldo C: Laparoscopic ovarian cystectomy of endometriomas does not affect the ovarian response to gonadotropin stimulation. *Fertil. Steril.* 2002;78:876–878

[29] Vercellini P, Aimi G, De Giorgi O, Maddalena S, Carinelli S, Crosignani PG. Is cystic ovarian endometriosis an asymmetric disease? *BJOG* 1998;105:1018-21.

[30] Esinler I, Bozdag G, Aybar F, Bayar U, Yarali H. Outcome of in vitro fertilization/ intracytoplasmic sperm injection after laparoscopic cystectomy for endometriomas. *Fertil. Steril.* 2006;85:1730–5.

[31] Yap C, Furness S, Farquhar C. Pre and post operative medical therapy for endometriosis. *Cochrane Database Syst. Rev.* 2004;3:CD003678.

In: In Vitro Fertilization
Editor: Samantha P. Steiger, pp. 131-163

ISBN 978-1-61209-961-3

Chapter VIII

Testis-Derived Male Germ-Line Stem Cells for Assisted Reproductive Technologies

Mukesh Kumar Gupta and Hoon Taek Lee*
Department of Animal Biotechnology, Bio-Organ Research Center/
Animal Resources Research Center, Konkuk University, Seoul, South Korea

Abstract

Importance of assisted reproductive technology (ART) is being increasingly realized due to progressively escalating cases of male infertility and diseases/treatments affecting spermatogenesis. Currently, sperm is the only choice to restore male fertility through ARTs. However, it may not be possible to retrieve sperm in all male infertility cases such as azoospermia or in prepubertal males who do not produce mature sperm. In such cases, testes-derived male germ-line stem (GS) cells and their in vivo counterpart, spermatogonial stem cells (SSC), have been envisaged as future therapeutic modality for the treatment of male infertility. Indeed, clinical trail of spermatogonial transplantation has already been conducted in both animal and human testes. Here, we describe the isolation, characterization and usage of SSC and GS cells in ARTs. We also discuss the current limitations in their usage and the possible measures to overcome them. Additionally, alternative methods of deriving sperm from somatic or stem cells have been discussed.

Introduction

Spermatogonial stem cells (SSCs) are a self-renewing population of testicular stem cells that are capable of differentiating into sperm throughout the adulthood. They lay the

* Correspondence: Hoon Taek Lee (htl3675@konkuk.ac.kr) / Mukesh Kumar Gupta (goops@konkuk.ac.kr); Fax: +82-2-4578488; Tel: +82-2-4503694.

foundation of spermatogenesis and fertility in males and can be cultured in vitro to generate male germ-line stem (GS) cells which can re-establish permanent spermatogenesis upon transplantation into recipient testes devoid of germ cells. In addition, under appropriate culture conditions, GS cells can acquire pluripotency to become multipotent GS (mGS; from neonatal testes) or multipotent adult GS (maGS; from adult testes) cells with the loss of spermatogenic properties (Guan et al., 2006; Kanatsu-Shinohara et al., 2004a). Since these testes-derived male germ-line stem cells can be cultured and genetically manipulated in vitro, they provide a powerful mean to correct male infertility, direct germ-line transmission of modified genomes, rapidly screen for germ cell-directed contraceptives, animal transgenesis, gene targeting through homologous recombination and gene trapping or enhancer trapping to define the gene function.

Usage and Significance of Testes-Derived Male Germ-Line Stem Cells

In Fertility Preservation and Restoration

Male infertility accounts for ~50% of total human infertility cases with ~20% as a sole cause and ~30% as a contributing cause (Hotaling and Walsh, 2009; Swan et al., 2000). It can be empirically treated with intracytoplasmic sperm injection (ICSI) as long as at least one motile sperm per oocyte is available. In cases wherein sperms are not available for ICSI or in patients who are expected to undergo chemotherapy for diseases such as cancer, testes-derived male germ-line stem cells can be envisaged as future therapeutic module (Fujita et al., 2005; Ogawa et al., 2000; Sadri-Ardekani et al., 2009). The usefulness of SSC in infertility treatment has already been well documented using mouse model system (Fujita et al., 2005; Ogawa et al., 2000). The proof-of-principle was provided by the restoration of fertility upon reciprocal SSC transplantation (SSCT) between infertile W locus and SCF mutant mice. Mutations in the dominant-white spotting (W; c-kit) and stem cell factor (SI; SCF) genes, which encode the transmembrane tyrosine kinase receptor and its ligand, respectively, are sterile because of the lack of differentiated germ cells or SSC but they become fertile upon reciprocal SSCT. It is therefore envisaged that cultivation of human SSC or GS cells may provide a tool to restore male fertility. It may have particular application in patients expecting to undergo radiotherapy or chemotherapies, for instance, after cancer therapies, which often disrupt spermatogenesis. Prior to the start of caner therapy, SSCs may be isolated from testicular biopsy samples and cryopreserved to restore the fertility by SSCT after successful completion of the cancer therapy. This approach is especially useful in pediatric patients, whose sperms are not available for preservation. Indeed, derivation of human SSCs from testicular biopsies and their cryopreservation has been successful and clinical trial of SSCT in human testis has already been conducted. Ginsberg and coworkers have been cryopreserving testicular tissue for young cancer patients since 2008 and have reported that this intervention was acceptable to parents and that testicular biopsies caused no acute adverse effects (Ginsberg et al., 2010). However, SSCT between two different individual has been skeptical in human due to ethical issues and likely histocompatibility problems because during SSCT,

SSC end up outside the Sertoli cell barrier (blood-testes-barrier; BTB) and hence, exposed to circulating immune system.

Since SSC and GS cells can be cryopreserved, they can also be used as a mean to preserve the genetic information of wild animal species in which sperms are difficult to preserve. Besides, it also allows the preservation of fertility in animals with defective or immature spermatogenesis.

In Transgenesis and Gene-Targeting

Testes-derived male germ-line stem cell has also added a new dimension to transgenesis and gene-targeting technologies. An ability to culture and genetically manipulate the SSC and GS cells in culture has lead to generation of transgenic animals by transplanting the genetically modified SSCs or GS cells into the testes of sires. This method is of particular use in animals such as pig and cattle in which other methods of transgenesis are not very efficient and authentic embryonic stem (ES) cells are not available for ES-mediated transgenesis. Furthermore, since SSC and GS cells can acquire pluripotency similar to that of ES cells, they are also capable of generating knockout animals in a manner similar to that of ES cells. Indeed, generation of knockout mice using mouse SSCs has been feasible after the successful establishment of protocols for the transplantation and long-term culture of these cells. Although not yet feasible, it may also be possible in future to produce transgenic animals by fertilizing an oocyte with a sperm that was in vitro differentiated from genetically modified SSC or GS cell.

In Regenerative Medicine and Stem Cell Research

Recent studies have demonstrated that SSC and GS cells can transition from being the stem cell-producing cells of spermatogenesis to being pluripotent mGS and maGS cells that can differentiate into derivatives of all three germ layers (Guan et al., 2006; Kanatsu-Shinohara et al., 2004a). Thus, they can not only serve as ethically acceptable sources for cell replacement therapies but also offer new possibilities for studying the mechanisms that regulate stem cell differentiation. The particular advantage in the use of mGS and maGS cells for cell therapies is that the cells can be taken from the patient, thereby evoking no immunological rejection. Besides, unlike induced pluripotent stem (iPS) cells, use of pluripotent cells generated from SSC eliminates the risks of insertional mutagenesis associated with integrated genes and obviates the need of exogeneous genes some of which are cancer causing.

SSCT also provide a useful method to study the biological effects of genes during sperm stem cell maturation. This method has been used to solve the old controversy regarding how spermatogenesis was regulated by androgen (Johnston et al., 2000). By SSCT of androgen-insensitive germ cell from mouse having testicular feminization syndrome to a normal mouse, it was shown that testosterone action was mediated via Sertoli cells and not germ cells (resulting in sperm formation). SSCT method has also been used to show that the timing of spermatogenesis is programmed by the genome of the germ cell and is apparently not under the influence of Sertoli cells. When germ cells were transplanted from a rat to a busulfan-treated mouse, the recipient could carry on both transplanted rat spermatogenesis and endogenous mouse spermatogenesis, each occurring at two different rates and each occurring at the characteristic rate of its donor-derived species (Franca et al., 1998).

Origin, Development and Self-Renewal of Testis-Derived Male Germ-Line Stem Cells

The SSCs arise from gonocytes in the postnatal testis, which in turn arise from primordial germ (PG) cells during fetal development. Thus, PG cells are the first germline cell in the embryo and therefore the SSC ancestor. They are first observed as a small cluster of Stella- and tissue nonspecific alkaline phosphatase (TNAP)-positive cells, adjacent to the extraembryonic ectoderm, in the epiblast stage embryo at about 7-7.25 days post coitum (dpc) in mouse. From here, PG cells proliferate and migrate to the genital ridge to associate with somatic gonadal precursor cells to form the gonad. Once within the gonad, they differentiate in a sex-specific manner, including a distinct program of proliferation and quiescence. At 12.5 dpc, Sry gene is expressed by Sertoli cells and the germ cells are committed to male lineage and spermatogenesis. Thus, if PG cells are removed before 12.5 dpc and mixed with 12.5 dpc female gential ridge cells, they enter the oogenesis pathway. On the other hand, if female PG cells are removed before 12.5 dpc and mixed with 12.5 dpc male genital-ridge, they are male committed. In the male genital ridge, PG cell become enclosed by the precursor Sertoli cells to form solid strands of cells called seminiferous cords which, later during the development, form a lumen to become seminiferous tubules. Within the seminiferous cords, PG cells substantial morphological and functional changes to become gonocytes which proliferate for a few days and then arrest at the G0/G1 phase of the cell cycle until around the time of birth, depending upon the species. In rats and mice, the gonocytes resume proliferation within a few days after birth and migrate from central position to the periphery in the seminiferous tubules to give rise to SSCs. During prepubertal development, the SSC population continues to expand and remains stable in adult animals. At the onset of reproductive age, SSCs initiate the first round of spermatogenesis to produce spermatogonia.

In adult mice, seven types of A spermatogonia (Asingle/As, Apaired/Apr, Aaligned/aal, and A1-4), intermediate spermatogonia (In) and type B spermatogonia (B) can be recognized (Figure 1). The Asingle spermatogonia are able to self-renew without further differentiation (and hence, assumed to be SSC), but can also produce differentiating daughter cells through many mitotic divisions, resulting in proliferative spermatogonia (Apr and Aal) and differentiated spermatogonia (A1-4, In and B). At the first division of As spermatogonia, Apr spermatogonia are connected by an intercellular bridge that is maintained between all cells in the germ cell cohort as the germ cells undergo mitosis and expand in number to form Aaligned spermatogonia. During epithelial stage VIII of spermatogenic cycle, almost all Aal spermatogonia, few Apr and very few As spermatogonia differentiate into A1 spermatogonia. These committed cells will then follow a strictly defined succession of steps, starting with six synchronized mitotic cycles (A1 to A4 cells, intermediate, and type B spermatogonia) before reaching the first meiotic stages. In human and monkeys, undifferentiated spermatogonia occur as Adark and Apale spermatogonia, with the Adark referred to as the reserve stem cells and the Apale being the renewing stem cells. However, there is limited information about how the Adark and Apale descriptions of nuclear morphology correlate with the clonal (As, Apr, and Aal), molecular, and functional descriptions of rodent SSCs. After Apale, spermatogonia differentiate into type B spermatogonia.

Two models have been proposed for SSC self-renewal:

1. A0/A1 or A0 Model

This model was first proposed by Clermont and Bustos-Obregon in 1968 (Clermont and Bustos-Obregon, 1968). According to this model, A0 spermatogonia are progenitor cells of the A1 spermatogonia and exist in very small number as quiescent cells. They have an indefinite or very slow cell cycle and divide only when there is an insult or injury to the tissue. The A1 cells are differentiating spermatogonia that divide to form A2-4 spermatogonia. The A4 spermatogonia can then divide to form either In spermatogonia or return to the A1 spermatogonia cell type to replenish them. If the testes encounter damages such as irradiation that prevents the replenishment of A1 spermatogonia by A4 spermatogonia, the A0 spermatogonia initiates cell division to replenish the A1 spermatogonia.

2. As model

This model was proposed by Huckins and Oakberg in 1971 (Huckins, 1971; Oakberg, 1971). According to this model, Asingle (As) spermatogonia can divide to either renew As spermatogonia or to become Apr spermatogonia (Figure 1).

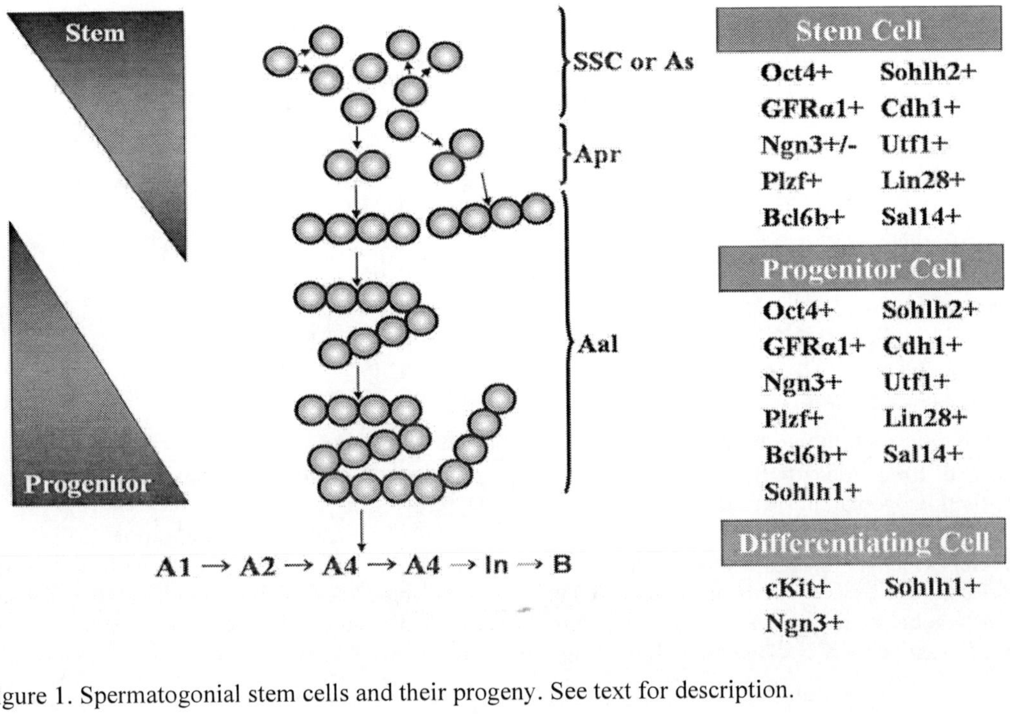

Figure 1. Spermatogonial stem cells and their progeny. See text for description.

Subsequently, Apr spermatogonia divide to form Aal spermatogonia that reach 4, 8, or 16 cells clone (termed Aal-4, Aal-8, and Aal-16, respectively). During stages VII-IX of the spermatogenic cycle, almost all Aal spermatogonia transform into A1 spermatogonia, a step that does not require mitosis, and then the A1 spermatogonia resume the cell cycle. Since differentiating Aal cells remain connected by intercellular bridges to form syncytial cysts of 2^n cells, As model assumes that the length of the cysts reflects their cell division history or lineage and cyst length reflects the extent of differentiation in a linear manner.

3. Extended as Model

In recent years, substantial progress has been made in identifying genes that are expressed in As cells and cysts of Apr and Aal. Using gene expression (GFRa1, PLZF, E-CAD and NGN3), cyst length, lineage analysis, and live imaging, Nakagawa et al., (2010) recently extended the long-held As model. According to this model, As cells does not represent the entire SSC. Instead "differentiating" spermatogonial cells can also act as "potential stem cells" - defined as cells that do not normally self-renew during steady-state spermatogenesis but nonetheless retain latent self-renewing potential. They found that GFRα1 and Ngn3 are expressed in minor and major subpopulations of the total As, Apr, and Aal population, respectively. The potential stem cells include not only the Ngn3+ As cells, but also Apr and Aal (either Ngn3+ or GFRα1+) cells. On the other hand, the population of GFRα1+ As cells, which is positioned at the top of both hierarchies, was best related to the "actual stem cells" that support normal steady-state spermatogenesis. Furthermore, only a part of the GFRα1+ As population persists for a long period to serve as functional stem cells, and a majority of this population does not self-renew continually and may act as "potential stem cells" as well. During differentiation, cells make a transition from GFRα1+→Ngn3+→A1 spermatogonia.

Table 1. Markers used to identify SSC and their progeny*

Cell Type	Marker
As and Apr	GFRα1
As, Apr, and Aal	Plzf, Oct4, Ngn3, Notch1, Sox3, c-Ret
A spermatogonia	Rbm
Spermatogonia	Ep-cam
Premeiotic germ cells	Stra8, EE2
Cells on basal membrane and interstitium	Cd9
Spermatogonia, spermatocytes, and round spermatids	GCNA1
Premeiotic spermatogonia and postmeiotic spermatids	Taf4B

*Adapted from "de Rooij, D. G., and Russell, L. D. (2000) All you wanted to know about spermatogonia but were afraid to ask. J. Androl. 21, 776–798."

Abbreviations: GFrα1: GDNF family receptor α1, Plzf: Promyelocytic leuchaemia zinc finger, Oct4:Octamer 4, Ngn3: Neurogenin 3, Sox3: SRY (sex determining region Y)-box 3, c-Ret: Rearranged during transformation / GDNF receptor, Rbm: RNA binding motif protein, Ep-cam: Epithelial cellular adhesion molecule, Stra8: Stimulated by retinoic acid gene 8, EE2: EE2 114 kDa antigen, GCNA1: Germ cell nuclear antigen 1, Taf4B: TATA box binding protein-associated factor 4B.

Cellular and Molecular Characteristics of SSC

The SSCs are rare cells and represent only a very small percentage of total cells in the mammalian testis. In mouse, there are about 10^8 cells in the testis and approx 2-3 x 10^4 are thought to be stem cells (Tegelenbosch and de Rooij, 1993). The SSC (As spermatogonia) constitute 10.6% of the undifferentiated spermatogonia, 1.25% of all spermatogonia, and 0.03% of all germ cells (Tegelenbosch and de Rooij, 1993). However, both the concentration and number of SSC vary with species (Orwig et al., 2002). For example, rat testis contains about 1 stem cell per 504 total cells (418.5 x 10^6 stem cells per testis) (Huckins, 1971).

Cellular Characteristics

SSCs occur as small round cells lining the periphery of the seminiferous tubules. Cytologically, As, Apr, and Aal spermatogonia could be differentiated from other testicular cell types based primarily on mottling of heterochromatin throughout the nucleus in the absence of heterochromatin lining the nuclear envelope. The As, Apr, and Aal spermatogonia can further be distinguished from each other based on the number of interconnecting cells (i.e. the length of the cyst), lineage analysis and live imaging (Figure 1). The A1 cells display finely granular chromatin throughout the nucleus and virtually no flakes of heterochromatin along the nuclear membrane. The A2 through A4 spermatogonia contain progressively more heterochromatin rimming the nucleus. On the other hand, In spermatogonia display flaky or shallow heterochromatin that completely rims the nucleus while Type B spermatogonia show rounded heterochromatin periodically along the nuclear envelope.

Expression of Cell Surface Markers

Cell surface proteins that are either exclusively expressed or are enriched on SSC compared to other testicular cell types provide a potential tool to identify and isolate the pure population of SSC from the testis. For example, thymus 1 (Thy1.2, CD90) protein were first identified as being expressed by SSCs compared to other germ cells in the testis of mice (Ryu et al., 2005). Unfortunately, although the expression of certain genes are restricted to As, Apr, and Aal spematogonia, there are no specific genes to distinguish SSCs (As spermatogonia) from their differentiated progeny (Apr and Aal spematogonia) and hence are not a clear phenotypic or molecular marker to identify SSCs. The expression of some markers is also not consistent across species. For example, Ep-cam is expressed on the surface of rat SSCs but not mouse (Nakagawa et al., 2010; Ryu et al., 2005). A list of molecules expressed on the surface of the SSCs is presented in Table 1. Among these surface molecules, α6/β1-integrin+, Thy-1+, CD9+ testicular cells are known to be enriched in SSC cells but are not a pure population of SSC. Thus, functional transplantation of marker-selected donor cells is the best assay to identify and validate undifferentiated SSC.

Expression of Transcription Factors

Loss-of function studies have revealed several important molecules required for the proliferation and biological function of SSCs. Since glial cell line-derive neurotrophic growth factor (GDNF) is an essential growth factor for self-renewal of SSCs, using the microarray-based gene expression profiling, Oately et al. (2007; 2006) have identified several genes regulated by the GDNF. They found that several transcription factors including Bcl6b (B cell CLL/lymphoma 6, member B), Etv5 (Ets variant gene 5; *Erm*) and Lhx1 (Lim homeobox protein 1) were involved in the regulation of SSCs self-renewal. Biological activity of these GDNF-regulated transcription factors to SSCs function was confirmed by functional transplantation. It was further demonstrated that GDNF regulate the expression of downstream Bcl6b, Etv5, and Lhx1, through the activation of Src family kinase signaling. SSCs also express Oct3/4, Sox2, Klf4, c-Myc and Lin28 which are pluripotency makers for ES cells and, upon exogenous introduction, can reprogram the somatic cell to iPS cells. Notably, Nanog, another important transcription factor for self-renewal of ES cell, is not expressed in the SSC. However, a recent report showed that SSC express Nanog upon acquisition of a pluripotency state as mGS or maGS cells.

SSC Niche

In the testes, SSCs are believed to reside within specialized microenvironments called 'niches', which regulates their specific properties including self-renewal, quiescence and the ability to differentiate into single or multiple lineages. The supporting cells within the niche provide a sheltering environment where stem cells can sequester differentiation stimuli, apoptotic stimuli, and other stimuli that would challenge the stem cell reserves (Watt and Hogan, 2000).The concept of niche was first proposed in 1978 by Schofield for haematopoietic stem cells (Schofield, 1978) and was later extended to all adult stem cells including the testes-derived male germ-line stem cells. However, in the mammalian testis, the anatomical site and the cells that compose the niche is controversial. Furthermore, little is known about the cellular, molecular and biochemical mechanisms that govern the establishment and maintenance of SSC niche.

Anatomical Location and Development of SSC Niche

Although exact location of SSC niche in mammalian testes remains a mystery, recent studies suggest that SSC niche including As spermatogonia and their direct descendants (Apr and Aal spermatogonia) are preferentially located in those areas of the seminiferous tubules that border on the interstitial tissue. Fewer of these cells are present in tubule areas directly bordering on another tubule. Yoshida et al. (2007) recently demonstrated that Apr and Aal spermatogonia (the direct descendents of SSC) develop preferentially in the area of the seminiferous tubules adjacent to the vasculature and interstitial cells.

The SSC niches are formed early during postnatal development when Sertoli cells start maturing. During the neonatal stage, the number of niches is likely determined by the number of SSCs. However, with age, the number and the activity of SSC decreases, possibly due to significant decrease in the production of GDNF by Sertoli cells (Ryu et al., 2005). Using 5-9 days old W/Wv mice as recipient to receive different ages of donor testicular cells, Shinohara et. al. (2001) showed that the proportion of SSCs in the total testis was larger when donor testicular cells were transplanted from day 5-12 old mice than from 14-20 weeks mice. Similarly, Zhang et al., (2006b) transplanted the SSCs from young, fertile male mice into the 1-year and 2-year atrophied testes of old males. They observed that 1-year-old testes were permissive for the regeneration of spermatogenesis, while the 2-year-old testes were not, suggesting a gradual change in the SSC microenvironment. However, in reciprocal transplantation experiments, colonization of young testes by 2-year-old SSCs was not as efficient as colonization by 1-year-old SSCs, indicating that stem cell intrinsic factors are also altered as the animal ages (Zhang et al., 2006b).

Cellular Composition of SSC Niche

The physical compartment of SSC location suggests that the somatic cells (Sertoli cells and peritubular myoid cells) and basement membrane of the seminiferous tubule participate as components of SSC niche. However, the interaction between Sertoli cell and SSC has been addressed more than basement membrane and SSC interaction. Emerging evidences further suggest that stimuli from the vascular network and interstitial cells in the testis might also be crucial for the SSC regulation and hence, may contribute to the SSC niche (Yoshida et al., 2007).

1. Sertoli Cells

Sertoli cells, which were first described by Enrico Sertoli in 1865, are somatic cells surrounding the germ cells within the seminiferous epithelium. They are large sized (75-100 μm) columnar shaped cells with a distinctive tripartite nucleolus in the nucleus and extend from the basement membrane of seminiferous epithelium to the lumen. Based on the spermatogenesis stage, Sertoli cells can be divided into two different morphologies: type A and type B. In type A Sertoli cells, mature spermatids reside within cytoplasmic crypts and are ready for release into the tubule lumen. However, in type B Sertoli cells, the cytoplasmic crypts are either barely observed or completely absent. The Sertoli cells are formed early in the embryonic development and start dividing and maturing at around 12.5 dpc in mice. During the pubertal stage of development, mature Sertoli cells stop dividing and start differentiating to form tight junctions and release nutrients for supporting the germ cell development. The proliferation and differentiation of Sertoli cells depends on hormonal regulation, especially by follicle stimulating hormone (FSH) released from the anterior pituitary. The number of mature Sertoli cells however, remains stable for the entire life of the mammal, and therefore their supportive capacity for germ cell development is determined at the beginning of puberty (Petersen and Soder, 2006).

Sertoli cells secrete several growth factors and hormones which influence cellular function, growth and differentiation at the molecular level through receptor-mediated signal transduction. The factors include insulin-like factors (IGFs), transforming growth factor α (TGFα), transforming growth factor β (TGFβ), fibroblast growth factor (FGF), neurotropins, basic fibroblast growth factor (bFGF or FGF2), epidermal growth factor (EGF) cytokines, kit ligand/stem cell factor (SCF), and GDNF. Among all these factors, GDNF is so far the only known paracrine factor in the testes specifically responsible for the maintenance and self-renewal of SSCs in vivo and in vitro (Kubota et al., 2004b; Meng et al., 2000). Other growth factors secreted by Sertoli cells, such as bFGF and EGF, while necessary for the SSC proliferation in vitro (Kubota et al., 2004b), do not appear to be sufficient for self-renewal in vivo. The general function of some of these factors and their specific function for testicular function are discussed below.

a. GDNF

GDNF is a distant member of the TGFβ superfamily, in which, with three other related molecules, it forms a subfamily called GDNF family ligands (GFLs). They all bind to and activate RET (rearranged during transfection) tyrosine kinase transmembrane receptor but require GDNF family receptor α:s (GFRαs) for ligand binding and Ret activation. In neuronal cells, GFLs also use neural cell adhesion receptor as an alternative signal transducing receptor (Sariola and Saarma, 2003). GDNF has been shown to be the most important regulator in the SSC self-renewal mechanism. In mice that overexpress human GDNF in their testes, the SSC number was dramatically increased, while GDNF knockout mice had depleted SSCs (Meng et al., 2000). On the other hand, GDNF+/- mice had reduced number of SSCs and increased apoptotic bodies in undifferentiated spermatogonia which illustrate the importance of GDNF concentration in maintaining the SSCs survival. Thus, GDNF is not only essential for SSC proliferation but also for the maintenance of SSC population.

b. Ets-Related Molecule (ERM)

ERM belonging to Ets transcription factor superfamily and is important for SSC self-renewal. Targeted disruption of Etv5 (Etv5-/-) results in normal testes histology at birth and completion of the first wave of spermatogenesis during juvenile life but, by 10 weeks of age, testes show Sertoli cell-only phenotype with complete disappearance of all germ cells (Chen et al., 2005). Although the exact mode of action is not known, knockout of ERM gene interfered with the expression of several downstream genes including GDNF and CXCL5 in Sertoli cells (Chen et al., 2005; Hess et al., 2006). Thus, ERM molecules are additionally believed to be important in creating the SSC niche, allowing for the rapid proliferation and growth of SSC in the basal compartment.

c. SCF

SCF, also known as kit ligand, is important for the PG cell viability and migration to the embryonic gonad. In c-kit mutant mice, most PG cells do not migrate to the genital ridge due to a mutation of the kit receptor that prevents kit ligand activation of the kit (Koshimizu et al., 1992). The kit expression is also important for spermatogonial differentiation from undifferentiated spermatogonia to differentiated spermatogonia (Schrans-Stassen et al., 1999). However, addition of kit ligand to in vitro culture medium did not increase the number of SSCs (Kanatsu-Shinohara et al., 2003). The expression of kit also varies between species and may play differential roles in the initiation of spermatogenesis. In rats, kit is expressed on undifferentiated spermatogonia before the postnatal stage but in neonates it is expressed only on the differentiated spermatocytes (Hamra et al., 2005). On the other hand, testes from day 1 mice did not stain for kit but its expression gradually increased after postnatal day 1.

d. Leukemia Inhibitor Factor (LIF)

LIF is a four-alpha-helix protein that contains three functional binding sites to interact with the receptor, gp130. It is a growth factor that is essential for the survival of different types of stem cells including GS cells from neonatal mouse testes (Kanatsu-Shinohara et al., 2004a). In mice testes, LIF is expressed in both Sertoli cells and peritubular myoid (PM) cells and may activate the JAK-STAT pathway to maintain SSCs population. It has been known that mice embryonic fibroblast cells (MEF) can secrete LIF to maintain ES cell survival. In experiments in which SSCs were co-cultured with MEF, the SSCs proliferated in the first seven days and then the cell number was maintained. Thus, LIF influence SSC survival rather than self-renewal and proliferation. Kanatsu-Shinohara et al., (2007) showed that addition of LIF to culture medium with or without GDNF did not affect the rate of proliferation but enhanced the colony formation in neonatal testis-derived GS cells.

e. FGF

Among several members of the FGF protein family, bFGF is the most studied FGF protein which is produced by Sertoli cells under the regulation of FSH. The receptor for bFGF is expressed in germ cells, Sertoli cells, Leydig cells, and PM cells. It has been suggested that bFGF mediates the interaction between these testicular cells. In mouse SSC culture, inclusion of bFGF to a serum free media was important for proliferation of SSCs (Kubota et al., 2003). However, it is not clear if bFGF acts directly on the SSCs or acts to stimulate the production of other factors by the feeder cells. In Sertoli cells, FGF2 also upregulates the expression of Etv5 in vitro, which is important for SSC renewal (Kubota et al., 2003; Yoon et al., 2009). Therefore, in addition to a direct effect of FGF2 on SSCs, an indirect paracrine effect of FGF2 on Sertoli cells appears possible.

f. IGFs

The IGFs are similar to insulin in their structure and include IGF-I and IGF-II. They stimulate DNA synthesis in proliferating Sertoli cells and influence the production of lactate and transferrin by the adult Sertoli cells. IGF-I not only acts on Sertoli cells themselves through autocrine mechanisms but also enhances the action of FSH on Sertoli cells. IT also regulate in vitro steroidogenesis in Leydig cells which thereby, suggest a regulatory loop between Sertoli cells and Leydig cells through IGF-1, although functional evidences for this regulatory loop has not been established.

g. TGF

TGF is a member of the EGF family and can locally interact with germ cells and peritubular cells. TGFβ has three isoforms, including TGFβ1, TGFβ2, and TGFβ3, which are all expressed by Sertoli cells. In the fetal rat testes, TGFβ1 inhibits cord formation and also antagonizes EGF function (Cupp et al., 1999). Furthermore, cultured Leydig cells treated with TGFβ1 results in inhibition of LH-induced testosterone production (Gautier et al., 1997). TGFβ1 and TGFβ2 expression is high in the prepubertal animal and then decrease to low levels in the adult. Interestingly, TGFβ3 has a transient increase at the onset of puberty but the functional significance of this increase is not known (Mullaney and Skinner, 1993).

2. Peritubular Myoid (PM) Cells

PM cells are embedded in the basement membrane of seminiferous tubules. Seminiferous tubules of large animals and primates has multiple layers of PM cells each of which is lined by basement membrane material and are separated from one another by type I collagen fibrils, elastin fibrils, and microfibrils. They are believed to secrete essential factors to influence the SSC niche but only a limited amount of information is available about the mechanisms regulating the function of PM cells. The PM cell androgen receptor specific knockout mice show dramatically reduced testicular size sperm production (Zhang et al., 2006a). A role for the PM cell product colony-stimulating factor 1 (Csf1) on SSC maintenance has also been suggested (Oatley et al., 2009). Csf1 was found to be expressed in interstitial Leydig and PM cells, whereas the Csf1 receptor (Csf1r) was highly enriched in Thy1+ cell fractions from pre-pubertal and adult mouse testes.

3. Basement Membrane of Seminiferous Tubules

The basement membrane is located between seminiferous epithelium and the PM cells as a thin zone of extracellular matrix composed of laminin, type IV collagen, heparan sulfate proteoglycan, and nidogen/entactin (Dym, 1994). In vitro experiments has shown that laminin and type IV collagen are produced by both Sertoli and PM cells while fibronectin is produced by PM cells alone (Richardson et al., 1995). The basement membrane is important for maintaining the columnar shape and polarity of Sertoli cells (Dym, 1994). Furthermore, α6-integrin, expressed by SSCs, can anchor with laminin to allow them to attach and grow. The basement membrane may also play an important role in the germ cell mobility during spermatogenesis and SSC proliferation during self-renewal (He et al., 2005; Kanatsu-Shinohara et al., 2006).

Regulation of SSC Niche

SSC self-renewal within the niche and their differentiation outside the niche is tightly regulated by both intrinsic gene expression within the SSC and extrinsic signals, including soluble factors and adhesion molecules, from the surrounding microenvironment. SSC-expressed genes such as Plzf, a transcriptional repressor protein, and Taf4b, a germ cell-specific component of the RNA polymerase complex, are considered to be essential for SSC self-renewal, whereas the transcription factors Sohlh1 and 2 appear to be crucial for spermatogonial differentiation (Figure 1). On the other hand, Sertoli cells produce growth factors that stimulate both self-renewal (GDNF, FGF2, ERM) and differentiation (activin A, BMP4, and SCF) of the SSCs. Additional factors that could link the SSC niche to the somatic cells outside the seminiferous tubules are Csf1, produced by Leydig cells that stimulate SSC proliferation and FSH that stimulates GDNF production by Sertoli cells. In addition, adhesion molecules that connect the SSCs to the basement membrane and cellular components of the interstitium between the seminiferous tubules are important regulators of the niche function.

1. Intrinsic Factors

a. Taf4b

Taf4b is a component of the RNA Polymerase II basal transcription apparatus and is germ cell specific (Falender et al., 2005). In mouse, it is expressed in gonocytes of the postnatal testes, and in spermatogonia and spermatids of the adult testes. It is not expressed in Sertoli cells. Taf4b knockout mice have normal testis histology at birth with normal completion of the first wave of spermatogenesis and transient fertility. However, the SSCs start to disappear as soon as 3 days after birth with progressive loss of the germ cells resulting in Sertoli cell-only seminiferous tubules and testicular atrophy after 12 weeks of age. However, taf4b -/- Sertoli cells support spermatogenesis of transplanted wild type spermatogonia (Falender et al., 2005). Thus, Taf4b is an SSC-intrinsic factor essential for the SSC self-renewal.

b. Plzf

Promyelocytic Leukaemia Zinc-Finger (Plzf) is a transcriptional repressor and is crucial for the regulation of SSC self-renewal. It inhibits stem cell differentiation and helps maintaining their presence in the niche possibly by repressing c-kit, which is a characteristic of spermatogonial differentiation (Filipponi et al., 2007). Thus, naturally occurring mutants lacking plzf (Luxoid) as well as experimentally created plzf knockout mice show progressive lose of spematogonia with increasing age (Buaas et al., 2004; Costoya et al., 2004). Undifferentiated spermatogonia isolated from plzf -/- mice also exhibit a marked increase in c-kit expression. Furthermore, the germ cells from the testes of Luxoid mutants cannot repopulate the testes of recipient W/Wv mice, suggesting that the defect is inherent to the SSCs.

2. Extrinsic Factors

Among all somatic cells, Sertoli cells appear to be the major contributors to SSC niche regulation by physically supporting the SSCs and providing them with growth factors. Besides, factors secreted by somatic cells outside the seminiferous tubules may also mediate their effect via Sertoli cells (Chen et al., 2005). The SSC niche regulation by Sertoli cells changes with age. During perinatal period of development, SSC self-renewal is mainly controlled by the GDNF while it is dependent on the ERM during the pubertal period (Chen et al., 2005; Hess et al., 2006; Meng et al., 2000). ERM-regulated pathways are coincident with the termination of Sertoli cell proliferation and commencement of the cycle of spermatogenesis, which is sustained by the same cell that regulates the stem cell niche (Hess et al., 2006).

a. ERM/Etv5 Transcription Factor

Etv5 (Ets Variant Gene 5) is a member of Pea3 group of the Ets family of proteins, which are characterized by a highly conserved DNA-binding ETS domain. It is expressed in both Sertoli cells and germ cells (Chen et al., 2005; Oatley et al., 2007) and plays an important role in balancing the SSC self-renewal and differentiation. Targeted disruption of the Etv5 (Etv5-/-) results in defective maintenance of the SSC pool without affecting the spermatogonial differentiation (Chen et al., 2005). Similar to Plzf-/- mice, Etv5-/- mice has normal testes histology at birth and complete the first wave of spermatogenesis during juvenile life. However, by 10 weeks of age they show Sertoli cell-only phenotype with complete disappearance of all germ cells due to a progressive loss of spermatogenesis (Chen et al., 2005). Although the exact mode of action is not known, analysis of Etv5-/-Sertoli cells detected a 9- to 25-fold reduction in several chemokines and a 10-fold reduction in matrix metalloproteinase-12 (MMP-12) expression which are important for stem cell recruitment, migration and homing. The expression of Etv5 in Sertoli cells is possibly regulated by local soluble factors as its expression was shown to be up-regulated by FGF2 and EGF but not by testosterone or FSH (Simon et al., 2007).

b. GDNF

GDNF is a member of the TGFβ superfamily that was originally identified as a survival factor for midbrain dopaminergic neurons (Lin et al., 1993) but has been shown to have several other function such as kidney morphogenesis (Sariola and Saarma, 2003), oocyte maturation (Linher et al., 2007) and ovarian tumorigenesis (Aravindakshan et al., 2006). In testis, GDNF is normally secreted from Sertoli cells and its receptors, GFRα1 (GDNF-family receptor α1) and Ret (rearranged during transformation), are expressed in undifferentiated spermatogonia (Meng et al., 2000; Yomogida et al., 2003). It plays a key role in determining the fate of SSCs (Hofmann et al., 2005; Kubota et al., 2004b; Meng et al., 2000). Overexpression of GDNF in mouse testes stimulated the self-renewal of SSC and blocked their differentiation (Meng et al., 2000; Yomogida et al., 2003). On the other hand, in the testes of mice with one GDNF-null allele, undifferentiated spermatogonia disappeared in older males and resulted in Sertoli cell-only seminiferous tubules (Meng et al., 2000). Exogenous supplementation of GDNF is therefore, considered essential for maintaining the self-renewal of SSC under in vitro conditions (He et al., 2008; Hofmann, 2008; Kubota et al., 2004a; b).

However, the regulatory signals that induce GDNF production and release have not yet been established. In neural cells, the induction of GDNF mRNA production and protein release is generally due to activation of the MEK/MAPK signaling pathway (Hisaoka et al., 2007), while transcription factor Pax2 plays an important role in GDNF expression in embryonic kidney. Deletion of the Hoxa11/Hoxc11/Hoxd11 gene cluster also results in the loss of GDNF expression in the embryonic kidney although these mice had normal expression of Pax2 (Wellik et al., 2002). Six2, a member of the Six family of homeobox containing transcription factors and Eya1 (mammalian ortholog of eyes absent in Drosophila) also activate GDNF gene expression in the embryonic kidney (Brodbeck et al., 2004). In testes, GDNF mRNA and protein have been localized in Sertoli cells (Meng et al., 2000), spermatogonia and spermatids (Yu et al., 2003) in the mouse. Similar results have also been reported for rats and humans (Yu et al., 2003). In Sertoli cells, the production of GDNF is likely under the influence of FSH, growth factors and cytokines secreted both locally and systemically (Simon et al., 2007; Tadokoro et al., 2002). Under in vitro conditions, GDNF production by Sertoli cells was also shown to be dependent on FGF2, TNFα and interleukin-1beta (Il-1β) (Simon et al., 2007). In Sertoli cell line TM4, FGF2 stimulated the expression of GDNF by 5-fold at 48 h after treatment while FSH stimulated the GDNF expression by 2-fold at 3-24 h after treatment (Simon et al., 2007). Stimulation of GDNF expression by FGF2 in TM4 cells was suppressed by pre-treatment of the cells with phosphatidyl inositol 3-kinase

(PI3K) inhibitor wortmannin and the mitogen-activated protein kinase (MAPK) signaling inhibitor PD98059. However, neither inhibitor alone or when added together completely abolished the FGF2-stimulated increase in the GDNF expression. This indicates that cellular mechanisms other than MAPK and PI3K pathways may also be involved in FGF2-mediated induction of GDNF expression. Interestingly, however, FGF2 knockout mouse are fertile (Ortega et al., 1998). It is also not clear how wortmannin or PD98059 affected FSH induction of GDNF in TM4 cells (Simon et al., 2007).

GDNF act downstream by activating multiple signaling pathways including PI3K and the Src family of tyrosine kinases. Bcl6b, a member of POZ (poxvirus and zincfinger) family of transcriptional repressors, is a verified target of GDNF signaling in the SSCs (Oatley et al., 2006).

I. Ras Signaling Pathway

Binding of GDNF with Rct rcccptor can activatc Ras signaling pathway. Upon ligand binding, Ret receptor autophosphorylates on its intracellular domain to serve as intracellular docking sites for different SH2-domain-containing proteins which, in turn can induce binding and activation of the adaptor proteins Shc and Grb2 to stimulate Ras/ERK1/2 pathway (He et al., 2008). This signaling cascade ultimately leads to the phosphorylation and activation of transcription factors such as Creb-1, Atf-1, and Crem-1 to up-regulate the transcription of the immediate-early gene c-fos, the cell cycle activator cyclin A, and cdk2, which all favors the G1/S cell cycle transition in GFRα-1 positive spermatogonia (Sunters et al., 2004).

ii. Src Signaling Pathway

SSCs also express several members (e.g. Src, Yes, Lyn and Fyn) of Src kinase family which co-precipitate with Ret after GDNF stimulation (Braydich-Stolle et al., 2007). Although the function of Src kinase family members overlap, it is believed that Src and Yes play a predominant role in the immediate response of SSCs to GDNF. Src activates a PI3K/Akt signaling pathway to stimulate the expression of N-myc which promotes SSC proliferation both in vivo (Lee et al., 2007; Oatley et al., 2007) and in vitro (Braydich-Stolle et al., 2007).

Table 2. Selection methods used for isolation of SSC populations from testes *

Selection method	Selection tool
Positive selection for protein expression	Cd9, integrin-α6, integrin-β, integrin-αV, Thy-1, Cd24
Negative selection for protein expression	c-kit, MHC1, LY6A, Cd34
Promoter-assisted expression of marker gene	Stra8, Oct4

*Adapted from "de Rooij, D. G., and Russell, L. D. (2000) All you wanted to know about spermatogonia but were afraid to ask. J. Androl. 21, 776–798."

Abbreviations: Thy-1: Thymocyte differentiation antigen 1 / Cd90, c-kit: v-kit Hardy-Zuckerman 4 feline sarcoma viral oncogene homolog, MHC1: Major histocompatibility complex class I molecule, LY6A: Lymphocyte antigen 6 complex, locus A, Stra8: Stimulated by retinoic acid gene 8, Oct4: Octamer 4.

iii. FGFR2 Signaling Pathway

FGFR2 is expressed in SSC and may play a role analogous to Ret in regulating SSC self-renewal and differentiation (Goriely et al., 2003). Besides, GDNF may also up-regulate the expression of FGFR2 in SSCs and thereby, increase their responsiveness to FGF2 for in vitro proliferation (Hofmann et al., 2005). Thus, GDNF and FGF2 are often used together to establish long-term cultures of gonocytes and SSCs (Kanatsu-Shinohara et al., 2003; Kubota et al., 2004b).

iv. B Cell CLL/Lymphoma 6, Member B (Bcl6b)

Bcl6b is a validated target of GDNF that was initially identified in SSCs by microarray analysis (Oatley et al., 2006). Targeted disruption of Bcl6b results in an increased incidence of Sertoli cell-only tubules in mice. Similarly, its inhibition of Bcl6b expression in in vitro cultured SSCs by RNA interference resulted in SSC depletion. Thus, Bcl6b has a critical role in SSC maintenance. Like N-Myc, Bcl6b is also a nuclear target of the Src signaling pathway (Oatley et al., 2007).

Isolation and Purification of SSC for Deriving GS Cells

Isolation of a purified population of SSCs is essential not only for their clinical transplantation but also for the derivation of GS cells that can be cultured in vitro for long-term either for clinical use or for understanding the regulatory mechanism of spermatogenesis and stem cell self-renewal. However, SSCs constitute only ~0.02-0.03% of all germ cell in adult testes and are heavily outnumbered by the differentiating spermatogonia, spermatocytes, spermatid and sperm that they produce. For research purpose, it is therefore, advantageous to isolate the SSC from the testes of young neonatal animals that do not contain the full complement of germ cells and hence, over 90% pure A spermatogonia could be prepared (Bellve et al., 1977). One can also use animal models in which undifferentiated spermatogonia are enriched experimentally. For example, in vitamin A-deficient rats and mice, spermatogenesis becomes arrested at the level of undifferentiated spermatogonia and therefore, 80–90% pure undifferentiated A spermatogonia can be prepared (van Pelt et al., 1996). Other models that show an arrest at about the same differentiation stages include cryptorchid mice (Shinohara et al., 2000) and irradiated rats (Shuttlesworth et al., 2000). However, in a clinical setting where we do not have the above options, an effective isolation method is required for the derivation and long-term culture of a pure population of SSC from a mixed testicular cell population. These methods are based on either positive or negative selection of SSCs with markers listed in Table 2. The heterogeneous testis cell suspension can be stained with a fluorescent-conjugated or magnetic bead-tagged antibody against SSC-specific cell surface antigen and positive cells can be fractionated by Fluorescence-activated cell sorting (FACS) or magnetic-assisted cell sorting (MACS). For example, Shinohara et al., (2000) tagged the total testicular cells with specific antibody against α6- and β1-integrin (receptors for laminin protein expressed in both mouse and rat SSC) to isolate α6- and β1-integrin-expressing cells by MACS. Transplantation assay revealed that these α6- and β1-integrin-expressing cells were enriched in SSC by approximately 5- to 7-fold compared with total testis cell population. Similarly, in rat, in vitro selection using laminin resulted in 8.5-fold enrichment (Orwig et al., 2002). In other studies, to improve the purity of isolated SSCs, a surface marker of hematopoietic stem cell, the glycosyl phosphatidylinositol (GPI)-anchored glycoprotein molecule Thy1 (Cd90), was used to select the SSCs. These Thy-1+ cell fraction were enriched approximately 30-fold compared with non-selected testicular cell population. Although expressed by both SSC and Apr spermatogonia, GFRα1 is also an adequate marker for purifying SSCs from testes (Buageaw et al., 2005). Using gravity sedimentation on a BSA gradient (STAPUT method) followed by magnetic beads isolation with a GFRα1 antibody, Hofmann et al., (2005) were able to isolate cell populations containing up to 98% SSCs. Thus, Thy1 (Cd90) and GFRα1 are currently the most commonly used antibodies for isolation of SSCs (Aponte et al., 2005). In human, G protein-coupled receptor 125 (GPR125) may be used as a marker for SSCs (Dym et al., 2009).

Unfortunately, the SSC in mammals has not been unequivocally identified through the use of germ cell-specific molecular markers or by other means although certain expression markers were helpful in isolating and enriching the SSC. The expression of some marker genes are restricted in proliferating spematogonia but none of them can specifically distinguish the SSCs (As spermagoonia) from their differentiated progenies (Apr and Aal spematogonia). Nonetheless, marker-selected cells are enriched in SSC compared to non-selected testicular cells. Use of a battery of molecular makers expressed on the surface of the SSCs (Table 3) may further increase the purity of SSC but it may reduce the total number of recovered cells. For example, α6/β1-integrin+, c-kit-, Thy1+, CD9+ testicular cells are enriched in authentic SSCs compared with non-selected putative SSC population. Mouse testicular cells characterized as side scatter (Bellve et al., 1977), α6-integrin+, β1-integrin+, Thy-1+, CD24+, CD9+, ckit–, αv-intergrin–, MHC-Ia/β2M–, sca-1–, CD34–, and cKit– have been sorted and shown to be enriched for SSC based on testicular colonization (Kanatsu-Shinohara et al., 2004b; Kubota et al., 2003; Shinohara et al., 2000). However, it should be noted that, these gene products are also expressed in different populations of differentiated testicular cells (Table 3) and, therefore, are not specific signatures for the SSC alone.

More commonly, SSCs are enriched by differential plating and laminin selection. This method does not require FACS or MACS and the isolated spermatogonia are greatly enriched in genetically modifiable SSCs that can develop into functional spermatozoa upon testicular transplantation (Hamra et al., 2005). The procedure is based on the principle that testicular somatic cells bind tightly to the plastic and collagen matrices on Petri dishes while spermatogonia and spermatocytes remain floating when they are cultured in a serum-containing medium. The collagen-non-binding testicular cells obtained using these procedures are thus ~97% pure spermatogenic cells from which putative SSC can be easily isolated by their short incubation on laminin-coated Petri dishes. The spermatogenic cells that bind to laminin matrix are more than 90% undifferentiated type A spermatogonia.

Isolation of SSC by Genetic Approaches

Genetic mouse models in which a reporter gene such as EGFP is expressed under the control of a promoter of SSC-marker gene provide an alternative approach for isolation of SSCs for research purposes (Table 2).

Table 3. Germ cell markers in rodent testes*

Marker	SSCT?	Type of germ cell								
		As	Apr	Aal	A1-4	In	B	Spc	Rs	Es
c-kit	No			√	√	√	√	√	√	
Ret	No	√	√	√						
Nanos2	Yes	√	√							
Pou5f1 (Oct4)	Yes	√	√	√						
Gfr-α1	Yes	√	√	√						
Thy1 (Cd60)	Yes	√	√	√						
Cdh1 (Cd324)	Yes	√	√	√						
Plzf	Yes	√	√	√						
Gpr125	Yes	√	√	√						
Ngn3	Yes	√	√	√				√		
Cd9	Yes	√	√	√	√	√				
β1-integrin (Cd29)	Yes	√	√	√	√	√	√			
α6-integrin (Cd49f)	Yes	√	√	√	√	√	√	√		
Nucleostemin	Yes	√	√	√	√	√	√	√		
Stra8	Yes	√	√	√	√	√	√	√	√	√
Egr3	Not Tested	√	√							
Nanos3	Not Tested	√	√	√						
Cd24	Not Tested	√	√	√						
Utf1	Not Tested	√	√	√						
Lin28 (Tex17)	Not Tested	√	√	√						
Sox-3	Not Tested	√	√	√						
Bcl6b	Not Tested	√	√	√						
Sohlh2	Not Tested	√	√	√						
Rbm	Not Tested	√	√	√	√					
Ep-Cam	Not Tested	√	√	√	√	√	√			
EE2 antigen	Not Tested	√	√	√	√	√	√	√		
Dazl	Not Tested	√	√	√	√	√	√	√		
Numb	Not Tested	√	√	√	√	√	√	√		
Gcna1	Not Tested	√	√	√	√	√	√	√	√	
Vasa (Mvh)	Not Tested	√	√	√	√	√	√	√	√	
Taf4b	Not Tested	√	√	√	√	√	√	√		√
Lrp4	Not Tested	√	√	√	√	√	√	√	√	√
Sohlh1	Not Tested			√	√	√	√	√		

*Adapted from Phillips et al., (2010) Spermatogonial stem cell regulation and spermatogenesis. Phil. Trans. R. Soc. B 365:1663-1678.

Abbreviations: As: A single spermatogonia; Apr: A paired spermatogonia; Aal: A aligned spermatogonia; A1–4: differentiating type A1 to A4 spermatogonia; In: intermediate type spermatogonia; B: type B spermatogonia; Spc: spermatocytes; Rs: round spermatids; Es: elongated spermatids;

SSCT?: Transplantable upon spermatogonial stem cell transplantation assay?

For example, Stra-8 (stimulated by retinoic acid-8), expressed by undifferentiated spermatogonia, including SSCs have been used to isolate SSC from adult mice (Giuili et al., 2002; Guan et al., 2006). Similarly, FACS-based isolation and transplantation of Oct4–

EGFP+/c-Kit- cells from the testis of transgenic mice expressing EGFP under the control of 18 kb promoter/enhancer fragment of the Oct4 gene had greater repopulation activity than Oct4-EGFP- or Oct-EGFP+/c-kit- cells (Ohbo et al., 2003). Neurogenin 3 (Ngn3) expressed by the earliest spermatogonia (Nakagawa et al., 2007; Yoshida et al., 2004) and Nanos2 expressed by SSC (Sada et al., 2009) have also been used to characterize SSC in mice. However, transplantation assays show that the isolated populations of SSCs were heterogeneous in their repopulation ability.

Derivation and Long-Term In Vitro Culture of GS Cells

Co-culture of putative SSC with various feeder cells such as STO and MEF have made it possible to culture SSCs for a long period of time, as was demonstrated by the SSCT assay. But it was Kanatsu-Shinohara et al., (Kanatsu-Shinohara et al., 2003) who first showed the long-term culture of SSC to derive the GS cells from neonatal mouse testes. The success of GS cell culture probably laid in the use of a proprietary culture medium of unknown composition and a combination of added growth factors, including GDNF (Kanatsu-Shinohara et al., 2004a). The GS cells expressed both spermatogonia- and pluripotent stem cell-marker genes and, upon testicular transplantation to infertile male, could initiate donor-derived spermatogenesis to produce fully functional spermatozoa that can contribute to live normal offspring. Subsequently, several research groups were successful in isolating the GS cells from neonatal as well as adult animals. Upon culture under appropriate conditions, GS cells formed colonies that usually comprised ~10 to 50 cells and proliferated with doubling time of 5 to 7 days. Several methodological variants have since then been described for the isolation and culture of GS cells. Basically, all currently used methods are based on supplementation of the culture medium with GDNF, growth factors such as FGF2 and LIF, vitamins and hormones. Both serum and serum-free methods have been developed (Hofmann et al., 2005; Kubota et al., 2004a; b). In some protocols, the cells are grown on feeder cells, either irradiated or mitomycin C-treated MEF or STO cells while in others, the cells are grown on laminin-coated dishes (Creemers et al., 2002; Kanatsu-Shinohara et al., 2006). Even a suspension culture system has been reported (Kanatsu-Shinohara et al., 2006).

Primary long-term cultures and immortalized cell lines of spermatogonia has also been established by gene modification to investigate the regulation of spermatogonial self-renewal and differentiation (Feng et al., 2002; Hofmann et al., 1994; Tascou et al., 2000). Pure SV40 large T immortalized spermatogonial cell lines were c-kit-negative and did not show any differentiation in vitro or in vivo. Similarly, a telomerase immortalized c-kit-positive spermatogonial line has also been established that was able to differentiate in vitro into spermatids. However, SSC activity by means of the SSCT assay was not tested for these cell lines.

In Vitro Spermatogenesis from Testes-Derived Male Germ-Line Stem Cells

Establishment of an in vitro spermatogenesis system would greatly enhance the clinical application of testes-derived male germ-line stem cells. It would also allow the study of stage-specific cellular interaction and molecular mechanisms underlying the specific gene regulation at different stages of spermatogenesis. It has been shown that somatic support cells can restrict the self-renewal of male germ-line stem cell and promote their differentiation (Kiger et al., 2000; Rassoulzadegan et al., 1993). For example, when mouse male germ cells were co-cultured on a Sertoli-like cell line, premeiotic germ cells underwent the meiotic and postmeiotic differentiation into haploid spermatids expressing the protamine gene (Rassoulzadegan et al., 1993). In another study, after 100 days in culture bovine spermatogonia were reported to differentiate into spermatocytes and spermatids based on various marker proteins (Izadyar et al., 2003). On the contrary, when isolated eel (Anguilla japonica) germ cells and somatic cells (mainly Sertoli cells) were co-cultured, the entire differentiation process from spermatogonia to spermatozoa was completed. These results imply that the initiation or completion of meiosis in normal male germ cells typically requires Sertoli cells or other somatic cells. However, in contrast with the mouse, primary spermatocytes in lower vertebrates such as amphibians (Abe, 1987) and fish (Sakai, 2002) differentiated into flagellated spermatids or functional sperm and did not require any supporting cells. The primary cultures of SSC or GS cells can also be stimulated to differentiate into pairs, chains, and germ cell colonies. However, the number of cells that progress through meiosis is generally negligible (Hamra et al., 2004; Izadyar et al., 2003; Kanatsu-Shinohara et al., 2003). Feng et al. (2002) reported the production of spermatocytes and spermatids from a stable mouse SSC line, though the fertilization potential of these cells was not tested. Unfortunately, a robust and reliable method for efficient generation of haploid germ cells from primary SSC cultures is not available for mammalian species including mouse and human.

A number of molecules have been shown to be involved in the differentiation of SSC and may hold the potential for future success in development an efficient in vitro spermatogenesis system. These include SCF/c-kit system, Dazl RNA binding protein, cyclin D2 and D3 and retinoic acid. In adult testis, c-kit is expressed in differentiating type A spermatogonia whereas Sertoli cells under FSH stimulation express its ligand, SCF. SCF/c-kit system upregulates cyclin D3 and promotes cell cycle progression in spermatogonia through a rapamycin-sensitive PI3K/p70 S6 kinase pathway (Feng et al., 2000). Mutations in the c-kit and the SCF genes have a variable effect on spermatogenesis, indicating that this system has a role at various stages in the spermatogenetic lineage. Dazl (deleted in azoospermia-like), on the other hand, is an RNA-binding protein and is expressed exclusively in spermatogonia. Its targeted disruption inhibited the differentiation of Aal spermatogonia into A1 (Schrans-Stassen et al., 2001) while transfection of ES cells with Daz gene family (Dazl, Daz and Boule) promoted their in vitro differentiation into germ cell lineage to form haploid gamete in both mouse (Yu et al., 2009) and human (Kee et al., 2009). However, it is not known if transfection of Daz would have same effect on in vitro differentiation of testes-derived male germ-line stem cells. In a more recently study, in vitro production of haploid sperm cells was shown to occur from male germ cells of fetal cattle when they were treated with retinoic acid (Dong et al., 2010).

There are several other factors that are involved in the differentiation of spermatogonia but need further investigation for their application in establishing a system for in vitro spermatogenesis. For example, cyclin-dependent kinases (cdks) and cyclins likely govern both the mitotic and meiotic divisions. The finding of null mice for cyclins D2 and D3 and Cdk4 suggest that cyclins D2 and D3 in combination with Cdk4, and possibly Cdk6, may regulate G1 progression and differentiation of spermatogonia (Sicinski et al., 1996; Tsutsui et al., 1999). Notch-1 signaling pathway may also function to maintain the proliferation of germ cells as they differentiate. Suppression of Notch-1 signaling using antibodies against Notch-1 or Jagged-2 led to maturation arrest in the rat testis (Hayashi et al., 2001) while addition of Jagged-1 in the culture media of freshly isolated SSCs increased their differentiation to Aal cells (Hofmann et al., 2005).

Haploid male germ cells have also been generated by differentiation of ES cells in mice (Geijsen et al., 2004; Nayernia et al., 2006; Toyooka et al., 2003) and humans (Kee et al., 2009). Two studies demonstrated that in vitro, ES cell-derived spermatids were competent to fertilize mouse eggs, generating blastocysts (Geijsen et al., 2004) and live progeny (Nayernia et al., 2006), respectively. However, because of the epigenetic reprogramming that occurs during in vivo germ cell development, the epigenetic regulation of in vitro gametogenesis must be carefully assessed before clinical applications ensue (Georgiou et al., 2007).

Derivation of Pluripotent Stem Cell from Testes

Recent studies have revealed that the SSC/GS cells can acquire pluripotency at the loss of spermatogenic potential when they are cultured under appropriate culture conditions. Kanatsu-Shinohara et al., (2004a) noticed that, when GS cells were continued to culture in vitro, a second cell type also appeared that could be expanded selectively under culture conditions used for ES cells (serum- and LIF- containing media lacking the GDNF). These cells, designated as mGS cells by the authors, were phenotypically similar to ES cells in colony morphology and doubling time, differentiated into various somatic cell types under conditions used to induce the differentiation of ES cells, produced teratoma when transplanted subcutaneously or into the seminiferous tubules of the testes and participated in normal embryonic development following injection into blastocysts. Thus, mGS cells were pluripotent and opened new opportunities for their use in regenerative medicine. Subsequently, Seandel et al., (2007) derived the ES-like colonies from GS cells using inactivated testicular stromal cells containing a mixture of Cd34+ peritubular cells, α smooth muscle actin (αSMA)-positive peritubular cells and Sertoli cell marker vimentin-positive cells as a feeder layer. However, Kanatsu-Shinohara et al., (2004a) failed to derive the mGS cells from adult testes. In 2006, Guan et al., (2006) reported a variant culture method that efficiently promoted ES cell-like cells formation from adult testes-derived cells. The SSCs were isolated from adult (4- to 6- weeks-old) mice transgenic for EGFP under Stra8 promoter (which is active in spermatogonia) and Rosa 26-LacZ. These mGS cells isolated from adult mouse testes were named maGS cells and were pluripotent. Similar to mGS cells, the maGS cells were able to spontaneously differentiate into derivatives of the three embryonic germ layers in vitro, to generate teratomas in immunodeficient mice and to contribute to the development of various organs when injected into an early blastocyst. The isolation of SSCs and derivation of maGS cells was not restricted to EGFP+ cells from the transgenic Stra8-EGFP/ROSA26-LacZ mouse (Stra8 mouse) alone. The maGS cell lines were also successfully derived from testes of four different strains of mice (FVB, C57BL/6, 129/Sv and the transgenic Stra8 mouse) by morphological criteria only. These results were also confirmed by other research groups including ours (Izadyar et al., 2008; Jung et al., 2010a; Oh et al., 2009; Seandel et al., 2007). It is however, not yet known whether SSCs are pluripotent themselves or in vitro generation of mGS and maGS cells resulted from genetic reprogramming of SSCs in culture. A recent study showed that a single SSC can dedifferentiate from a highly lineage-specified state to a pluripotent state (Kanatsu-Shinohara et al., 2008). This demonstrates that germ-line lineage cells probably retain the potential to generate pluripotent cells when they are cultured under appropriate culture conditions. However, the mechanism regulating the conversion of GS into mGS or maGS cells remains elusive.

Table 4. Differential characteristics of GS and mGS/maGS cells

Characteristics	GS Cell	maGS Cell
Cellular Proliferation	Slow; small-sized colony	Fast, bigger-sized colony
Doubling time	4-6 days	2-3 days
Effect of Serum on cellular proliferation	Detrimental	Beneficial
DNA methylation of imprinted genes (Peg1, Peg3, Meg3, Igf2-H19, Dio-Dlk1, Gnas)	Similar to sperm	Intermediate between GS and ES cell
Expression of Let-7 miRNA	High	Low
Transplantation in nude mice	No tumor	Tumor/teratoma
Testicular transplantation in W/Wv mice	Homing and spermatogenesis	Tumor/teratoma

Table 5. Summary of genes associated with GS and mGS/maGS cells

Cell type	Gene symbol
SSC and GS cell	Plzf (Zbtb 16), Ngn3 (Neurog3), GFRα1, Ret, Utp14b (jsd), Oct3/4 (Pou5f1), Bcl6b, Etv5 (ERM), Lhx1, Nanos2, Cd9, Dazl, Ep-cam, α6-integrin, β1-integrin, c-Ret, Rex1, Stra8.
mGS and maGS cells	Cd9, Dazl, Ep-cam, α6-integrin, β1-integrin, c-Ret, Rex1, Stra8, Klf4, Nanog, Sox2, Myc, Oct3/4 (Pou5f1), Plzf, SSEA-1.
ES cells	Cd9, Ep-cam, c-Ret, Rex1, Stra8, Klf4, Nanog, Sox2, Myc, Oct3/4 (Pou5f1), SSEA-1.

Characterization of Testes-Derived Stem Cells

The testes-derived male germ-line stem cells can be characterized by their morphology, culture characteristics, alkaline phosphatase (AP) activity and the expression of SSC- (for GS cells) and ES cell- (for mGS and maGS cells) marker genes and proteins (Tables 3, 4 and 5). Unlike GS cells, mGS and maGS cells form tightly packed colonies that generally appear within 10-15 days after initiation of the culture and morphologically resembled ES cell colonies that can be successfully propagated at a dilution of 1:3 to 1:6 every 3-4 days. The colonies are strongly positive for AP activity and show positive expression for markers expressed by ES (e.g. Oct4, Nanog, Cd9, Rex1) and GS (e.g. Stra8, Cd9, b1-integrin, a6-integrin, Ret) cells. The expression of these marker genes are maintained even after long-term culture. The colonies also show high expression of transcription factors (e.g. Oct4 and Nanog) and cell surface marker (SSEA1 and CD90 (Thy-1)) proteins in similar to ES cells (Table 5). A final confirmation can be done by SSCT assay to confirm the initiation of spermatogenesis by GS cells and formation of teratoma by mGS and maGS cells. The authenticity of mGS and maGS cells can further be verified by tetrapoloid complementation assay or by chimera formation through blastocyst injection to confirm their contribution to normal embryonic development.

The pluripotent mGS and maGS cells are also different from GS cell in several other aspects (Table 4). First, FBS does not favor SSC self-renewal in culture while it is not detrimental to maGS cell proliferation. Second, gene expression profiling of mGS and maGS cells is similar to that of ES cells. The mGS and maGS cells express a set of specific pluripotentcy marker genes including Oct3/4, Sox2 and Nanog. However, AP activity and the expression of pluripotency markers are reported to be low or absent in SSC clumps and cannot be identified in gonocytes and undifferentiated spermatogonia of postnatal mouse testes. Third, mGS and maGS cells do not have spermatogenic potential but produce teratoma when transplanted into the seminiferous tubules. Finally, GS cells show androgenetic genomic imprinting of SSC but undergo changes in DNA methylation pattern during their conversion to mGS (Kanatsu-Shinohara et al., 2004a) or maGS (Zechner et al., 2009) cells. However, the changes in DNA methylation pattern is incomplete and does not completely resemble the hemizygotic genomic imprinting pattern of ES or somatic cells. Zechner et al., (2009) showed that DNA methylation pattern of maGS cells resembled male ES cells more closely than that of mGS cells.

The mGS and maGS cells originate from the cultured GS cells themselves at a low frequency and are not some leftover of earlier type of germ cells (de Rooij, 2006; Kanatsu-Shinohara et al., 2004a; Ko et al., 2009). During this conversion, the androgenetic genomic imprinting in GS cells also changes to ES cell-like pattern in mGS or maGS cells (Kanatsu-Shinohara et al., 2004a; Zechner et al., 2009). Recently, we showed that mouse maGS cells are epigenetically stable for DNA methylation at imprinted *Igf2-H19* gene cluster during in vitro culture and differentiation (Oh et al., 2009) but re-acquire GS cell-like growth and differentiation characteristics with altered DNA methylation pattern when they are re-cultured in the GS-like conditions (Jung et al., 2010a). Thus, at any particular time point, *in vitro* cultured GS cells may contain some contaminating mGS or maGS cells which may produce teratoma instead of initiating spermatogenesis upon their transplantation into recipient testis (Guan et al., 2006; Jung et al., 2010a; Kanatsu-Shinohara et al., 2004a). Consequently, a molecular marker that can distinguish GS cells from mGS or maGS cells would be of potential value in both clinical and experimental research settings. We recently show that GS cells and maGS cells show differential expression of Let-7, miR-294 and imprinted miRNAs that can be used as a miRNA signature for their identification before research or clinical application (Jung et al., 2010a; Jung et al., 2010b). Thus, prior to SSCT, putative GS/maGS colonies may be screened for the expression levels of Let-7 and miR-294 and imprinting status of imprinted miRNAs by individually picking few cells from each individual colony and then be compared with those of sperm and ES cell controls. Low level of Let-7 and high level of miR-294 comparable to those of ES cells would suggest the presence of maGS cells while miRNA expression levels comparable to those of sperm would suggest that the colony originated from GS cells. Similarly, an androgenetic imprinting status comparable to those of sperm would suggest that the colony originated from GS cells. If necessary, the screened colonies may be expanded and further analyzed for full miRNA profile by miRNA micro-array analysis. The maGS cells would be expected to shown micro-array profile similar to those of ES cells (Zovoilis et al., 2008).

Spermatogonial Stem Cell Transplantation (SSCT)

The restoration of fertility in an infertile animal upon SSCT is the most solid proof of the GS cells' authenticity. This technique was pioneered in the laboratory of Ralph Brinster in 1994 (Brinster and Avarbock, 1994; Brinster and Zimmermann, 1994) and was proven to be a technological breakthrough in studying the biology of the testes-derived male germ-line stem cells and its microenvironment, the SSC niche (Brinster, 2002). In its initial days, SSCT involved the injection of a testicular cell suspension from a fertile donor into the testis of an infertile recipient. However, in recent days, its use has been extended as an assay to provide evidence that the cells in a suspension are SSCs. The SSCT assay system involve the injection of putative SSC population of donor into the seminiferous tubules of a recipient in which endogenous germ cells have been depleted either by treatment with chemotoxic drug (e.g., busulfan), irradiation, genetic modification (e.g., W/Wv mutant males) or are naturally depleted (e.g., Vitamin A deficiency, cryptorchism). The method involves following steps:

1. Preparation of Recipient Testis

To enable the evaluation of the success of the transplantation, the recipient testis should have no or negligible endogenous spermatogenesis. Such empty seminiferous tubule, having little or no germ cells, also provide a more favorable condition for homing of the donor SSC into the recipient testis. Thus, in a research or experimental set up for verifying the authenticity of putative SSC, recipient testis are depleted of spermatogenesis using chemical agents such as busulfan which is cytotoxic to germ cells (Brinster and Avarbock, 1994; Brinster and Zimmermann, 1994). However, busulfan is also toxic to bone marrow cells and therefore, the dose must be tested to determine if a particular strain or animal species will tolerate the injected dose while ensuing the cell loss. Moreover, it is likely that busulfan may not destroy all SCC within the recipient testis and, with time, there will be both transplanted and re-initiated endogenous spermatogenesis. In the occurrence of this event, a donor marker is needed to distinguish between the two types of spermatogenesis. Thus, donor cells are usually labeled with exogenous transgenes such as EGFP or LacZ gene encoding for β-galactosidase. In such cases, donor-derived spermatogenesis can be distinguished from endogenous spermatogenesis of recipient testis by visualizing the green florescent of EGFP under UV or assaying the enzyme activity of LacZ as a blue reaction product with the substrate X-gal. Since this approach require the use of a transgenic donor animal or in vitro genetic manipulation of donor cells prior to SSCT, it may not always be feasible. An alternative approach is to use the recipient testes of genetically sterile male whose somatic cells are capable of supporting spermatogenesis but cannot produce differentiating germ cells (Brinster and Avarbock, 1994). One such example is homozygous dominant white spotted mutant (W/Wv) mouse whose germ cells lack the functional c-Kit receptor and therefore, do not have endogenous spermatogenesis (Brinster and Zimmermann, 1994). Thus, any active spermatogenesis in these mice is likely to be from the donor-derived SSC only. Of note, such manipulations are cannot be performed in a clinical settings.

2. Preparation of Donor Cells

Donor cells are prepared as a single-cell suspension with a cell concentration of ~ 5×10^7 cells/ml to avoid their clumping and thereby, clogging of the injection micropipette during the injection process. The prepared donor cell suspension can then be microinjected into one of three sites of a recipient testis: i) into the lumen of seminiferous tubules using a micromanipulator; ii) into the rete-testis through the testis capsule by hand or micromanipulator; iii) into the rete-testis through the bundle of efferent ducts. The most widely used method involves inserting a needle through the efferent ductules outside of the testis and passing the needle into the rete-testis. The micropipet is hand-held and pressure is created manually using a 1-mL syringe connected to the micropipette to fill 30-100% of all seminiferous tubule in the recipient testis. A dye such as trypan blue can be microinjected along with the cells to monitor the extent of filling of seminiferous tubules.

3. Evaluating the Success of SSCT

Following SSCT, the SSC moves to the base of the tubule through Sertoli-Sertoli tight junctions to reside in their normal position along the tunica propria by unknown mechanisms and create normal seminiferous tubule architecture with stem cell division from the basal compartment to more mature cells near the lumen. Formation of spermatogonia, spermatocyte and sperm occur after ~2 month in mice. Spermatogenesis is initially confined to small regions within each seminiferous tubule and then expands in both directions along the tubule at a rate of over 50 μm/day. About 30% of testis can be colonized 3 months after SSCT and at least some sperms would be capable of fertilizing eggs and producing offspring (Brinster and Avarbock, 1994). Thus, the authenticity of SSC in the donor cells can be verified by allowing the donor cells to colonize the recipient testis for periods of several months (depending on the species) following which recipient males can be bred to determine if there are any donor-derived offspring. If EGFP or LacZ labeled donor cells were used for SSCT, authenticity of

SSC can be verified at an earlier time by histologically or histochemically examining the testis for the EGFP or β-galactosidase activity or by examining the epididymis for the presence of sperm.

Xenogenic SSCT

SSCT can be used to transfer testicular stem cells from one animal to another of the same species (referred to as syngeneic transplants) and sometimes to an animal of a different species (referred to as xenogeneic transplants). Thus, in the absence of recipient testis from same species, it is possible to perform SSCT assay using the immuno-compromised or immuno-deficient recipient testis from a related or even non-related species. Because immuno-compromised or immuno-deficient recipient animal do not mount an immune response against foreign cells, exogenous SSC will colonize the seminiferous tubules, and cell rejection will not occur. The success of xenogenic SSCT however, varies with the phylogenic distance between the two species. While Rat-to-Mouse SSCT is relatively successful, Hamster-to-Mouse SSCT is very difficult. Moreover, Pig/Horse/Bull/Dog/Rabbit-to-Mouse SSCT resulted in some seeding of the transplanted spermatogonia but little to no development was seen beyond the spermatogonial phase of spermatogenesis. The Human-to-Mouse SSCT was unsuccessful. The precise reason for low success or failure of xenogenic SSCT is not fully understood but it appears that somatic cell of recipient perhaps do not tolerate or facilitate the development of germ cells from another species. Furthermore, the timing of germ cell development is different in donor and recipient. The cycle exhibited by the Sertoli cells in one species may not match that of another species with a markedly different cycle length.

Conclusion

Testes-derived male germ-line stem cells have shown promising results in animal models and thus, have potential as a future therapeutic modality for infertility in human.

References

Abe, S. (1987) Differentiation of spermatogenic cells from vertebrates in vitro. *Int. Rev. Cytol.* 109:159-209.

Aponte, P.M., van Bragt, M.P., de Rooij, D.G., and van Pelt, A.M. (2005) Spermatogonial stem cells: characteristics and experimental possibilities. *Apmis* 113:727-742.

Aravindakshan, J., Chen, X.L., and Sairam, M.R. (2006) Age-dependent bimodal GDNF regulation during ovarian tumorigenesis in follitropin receptor mutant mice. *Biochem. Biophys. Res. Commun.* 351:507-513.

Bellve, A.R., Cavicchia, J.C., Millette, C.F., O'Brien, D.A., Bhatnagar, Y.M., and Dym, M. (1977) Spermatogenic cells of the prepuberal mouse. Isolation and morphological characterization. *J. Cell Biol.* 74:68-85.

Braydich-Stolle, L., Kostereva, N., Dym, M., and Hofmann, M.C. (2007) Role of Src family kinases and N-Myc in spermatogonial stem cell proliferation. *Dev. Biol.* 304:34-45.

Brinster, R.L. (2002) Germline stem cell transplantation and transgenesis. *Science* 296:2174-2176.

Brinster, R.L., and Avarbock, M.R. (1994) Germline transmission of donor haplotype following spermatogonial transplantation. *Proc. Natl. Acad. Sci. USA* 91:11303-11307.

Brinster, R.L., and Zimmermann, J.W. (1994) Spermatogenesis following male germ-cell transplantation. *Proc. Natl. Acad. Sci. USA* 91:11298-11302.

Brodbeck, S., Besenbeck, B., and Englert, C. (2004) The transcription factor Six2 activates expression of the Gdnf gene as well as its own promoter. *Mech. Dev.* 121:1211-1222.

Buaas, F.W., Kirsh, A.L., Sharma, M., McLean, D.J., Morris, J.L., Griswold, M.D., de Rooij, D.G., and Braun, R.E. (2004) Plzf is required in adult male germ cells for stem cell self-renewal. *Nat. Genet.* 36:647-652.

Buageaw, A., Sukhwani, M., Ben-Yehudah, A., Ehmcke, J., Rawe, V.Y., Pholpramool, C., Orwig, K.E., and Schlatt, S. (2005) GDNF family receptor alpha1 phenotype of spermatogonial stem cells in immature mouse testes. *Biol. Reprod.* 73:1011-1016.

Chen, C., Ouyang, W., Grigura, V., Zhou, Q., Carnes, K., Lim, H., Zhao, G.Q., Arber, S., Kurpios, N., Murphy, T.L., Cheng, A.M., Hassell, J.A., Chandrashekar, V., Hofmann, M.C., Hess, R.A., and Murphy, K.M. (2005) ERM is required for transcriptional control of the spermatogonial stem cell niche. *Nature* 436:1030-1034.

Clermont, Y., and Bustos-Obregon, E. (1968) Re-examination of spermatogonial renewal in the rat by means of seminiferous tubules mounted "in toto". *Am. J. Anat.* 122:237-247.

Costoya, J.A., Hobbs, R.M., Barna, M., Cattoretti, G., Manova, K., Sukhwani, M., Orwig, K.E., Wolgemuth, D.J., and Pandolfi, P.P. (2004) Essential role of Plzf in maintenance of spermatogonial stem cells. *Nat. Genet.* 36:653-659.

Creemers, L.B., den Ouden, K., van Pelt, A.M., and de Rooij, D.G. (2002) Maintenance of adult mouse type A spermatogonia in vitro: influence of serum and growth factors and comparison with prepubertal spermatogonial cell culture. *Reproduction* 124:791-799.

Cupp, A.S., Kim, G., and Skinner, M.K. (1999) Expression and action of transforming growth factor beta (TGFbeta1, TGFbeta2, and TGFbeta3) during embryonic rat testis development. *Biol. Reprod.* 60:1304-1313.

de Rooij, D.G. (2006) Rapid expansion of the spermatogonial stem cell tool box. *Proc. Natl. Acad. Sci. USA* 103:7939-7940.

Dong, W.Z., Hua, J.L., Shen, W.Z., and Dou, Z.Y. (2010) In vitro production of haploid sperm cells from male germ cells of foetal cattle. *Anim. Reprod. Sci.* 118:103-109.

Dym, M. (1994) Basement membrane regulation of Sertoli cells. *Endocr. Rev.* 15:102-115.

Dym, M., He, Z., Jiang, J., Pant, D., and Kokkinaki, M. (2009) Spermatogonial stem cells: unlimited potential. *Reprod. Fertil. Dev.* 21:15-21.

Falender, A.E., Freiman, R.N., Geles, K.G., Lo, K.C., Hwang, K., Lamb, D.J., Morris, P.L., Tjian, R., and Richards, J.S. (2005) Maintenance of spermatogenesis requires TAF4b, a gonad-specific subunit of TFIID. *Genes. Dev.* 19:794-803.

Feng, L.X., Chen, Y., Dettin, L., Pera, R.A., Herr, J.C., Goldberg, E., and Dym, M. (2002) Generation and in vitro differentiation of a spermatogonial cell line. *Science* 297:392-395.

Feng, L.X., Ravindranath, N., and Dym, M. (2000) Stem cell factor/c-kit up-regulates cyclin D3 and promotes cell cycle progression via the phosphoinositide 3-kinase/p70 S6 kinase pathway in spermatogonia. *J. Biol. Chem.* 275:25572-25576.

Filipponi, D., Hobbs, R.M., Ottolenghi, S., Rossi, P., Jannini, E.A., Pandolfi, P.P., and Dolci, S. (2007) Repression of kit expression by Plzf in germ cells. *Mol. Cell Biol.* 27:6770-6781.

Franca, L.R., Ogawa, T., Avarbock, M.R., Brinster, R.L., and Russell, L.D. (1998) Germ cell genotype controls cell cycle during spermatogenesis in the rat. *Biol. Reprod.* 59:1371-1377.

Fujita, K., Ohta, H., Tsujimura, A., Takao, T., Miyagawa, Y., Takada, S., Matsumiya, K., Wakayama, T., and Okuyama, A. (2005) Transplantation of spermatogonial stem cells isolated from leukemic mice restores fertility without inducing leukemia. *J. Clin. Invest.* 115:1855-1861.

Gautier, C., Levacher, C., Saez, J.M., and Habert, R. (1997) Transforming growth factor beta1 inhibits steroidogenesis in dispersed fetal testicular cells in culture. *Mol. Cell Endocrinol.* 131:21-30.

Geijsen, N., Horoschak, M., Kim, K., Gribnau, J., Eggan, K., and Daley, G.Q. (2004) Derivation of embryonic germ cells and male gametes from embryonic stem cells. *Nature* 427:148-154.

Georgiou, I., Pardalidis, N., Giannakis, D., Saito, M., Watanabe, T., Tsounapi, P., Loutradis, D., Kanakas, N., Karagiannis, A., Baltogiannis, D., Giotitsas, N., Miyagawa, I., and Sofikitis, N. (2007) In vitro spermatogenesis as a method to bypass pre-meiotic or post-meiotic barriers blocking the spermatogenetic process: genetic and epigenetic implications in assisted reproductive technology. *Andrologia* 39:159-176.

Ginsberg, J.P., Carlson, C.A., Lin, K., Hobbie, W.L., Wigo, E., Wu, X., Brinster, R.L., and Kolon, T.F. (2010) An experimental protocol for fertility preservation in prepubertal boys recently diagnosed with cancer: a report of acceptability and safety. *Hum. Reprod.* 25:37-41.

Giuili, G., Tomljenovic, A., Labrecque, N., Oulad-Abdelghani, M., Rassoulzadegan, M., and Cuzin, F. (2002) Murine spermatogonial stem cells: targeted transgene expression and purification in an active state. *EMBO Rep.* 3:753-759.

Goriely, A., McVean, G.A., Rojmyr, M., Ingemarsson, B., and Wilkie, A.O. (2003) Evidence for selective advantage of pathogenic FGFR2 mutations in the male germ line. *Science* 301:643-646.

Guan, K., Nayernia, K., Maier, L.S., Wagner, S., Dressel, R., Lee, J.H., Nolte, J., Wolf, F., Li, M., Engel, W., and Hasenfuss, G. (2006) Pluripotency of spermatogonial stem cells from adult mouse testis. *Nature* 440:1199-1203.

Hamra, F.K., Chapman, K.M., Nguyen, D.M., Williams-Stephens, A.A., Hammer, R.E., and Garbers, D.L. (2005) Self renewal, expansion, and transfection of rat spermatogonial stem cells in culture. *Proc. Natl. Acad. Sci. USA* 102:17430-17435.

Hamra, F.K., Schultz, N., Chapman, K.M., Grellhesl, D.M., Cronkhite, J.T., Hammer, R.E., and Garbers, D.L. (2004) Defining the spermatogonial stem cell. *Dev. Biol.* 269:393-410.

Hayashi, T., Kageyama, Y., Ishizaka, K., Xia, G., Kihara, K., and Oshima, H. (2001) Requirement of Notch 1 and its ligand jagged 2 expressions for spermatogenesis in rat and human testes. *J. Androl.* 22:999-1011.

He, Z., Feng, L., Zhang, X., Geng, Y., Parodi, D.A., Suarez-Quian, C., and Dym, M. (2005) Expression of Col1a1, Col1a2 and procollagen I in germ cells of immature and adult mouse testis. *Reproduction* 130:333-341.

He, Z., Jiang, J., Kokkinaki, M., Golestaneh, N., Hofmann, M.C., and Dym, M. (2008) Gdnf upregulates c-Fos transcription via the Ras/Erk1/2 pathway to promote mouse spermatogonial stem cell proliferation. *Stem Cells* 26:266-278.

Hess, R.A., Cooke, P.S., Hofmann, M.C., and Murphy, K.M. (2006) Mechanistic insights into the regulation of the spermatogonial stem cell niche. *Cell Cycle* 5:1164-1170.

Hisaoka, K., Takebayashi, M., Tsuchioka, M., Maeda, N., Nakata, Y., and Yamawaki, S. (2007) Antidepressants increase glial cell line-derived neurotrophic factor production through monoamine-independent activation of protein tyrosine kinase and extracellular signal-regulated kinase in glial cells. *J. Pharmacol. Exp. Ther.* 321:148-157.

Hofmann, M.C. (2008) Gdnf signaling pathways within the mammalian spermatogonial stem cell niche. *Mol. Cell Endocrinol.* 288:95-103.

Hofmann, M.C., Braydich-Stolle, L., and Dym, M. (2005) Isolation of male germ-line stem cells; influence of GDNF. *Dev. Biol.* 279:114-124.

Hofmann, M.C., Hess, R.A., Goldberg, E., and Millan, J.L. (1994) Immortalized germ cells undergo meiosis in vitro. *Proc. Natl. Acad. Sci. USA* 91:5533-5537.

Hotaling, J.M., and Walsh, T.J. (2009) Male infertility: a risk factor for testicular cancer. *Nat. Rev. Urol.* 6:550-556.

Huckins, C. (1971) The spermatogonial stem cell population in adult rats. I. Their morphology, proliferation and maturation. *Anat. Rec.* 169:533-557.

Izadyar, F., Den Ouden, K., Creemers, L.B., Posthuma, G., Parvinen, M., and De Rooij, D.G. (2003) Proliferation and differentiation of bovine type A spermatogonia during long-term culture. *Biol. Reprod.* 68:272-281.

Izadyar, F., Pau, F., Marh, J., Slepko, N., Wang, T., Gonzalez, R., Ramos, T., Howerton, K., Sayre, C., and Silva, F. (2008) Generation of multipotent cell lines from a distinct population of male germ line stem cells. *Reproduction* 135:771-784.

Johnston, D.S., Russell, L.D., and Griswold, M.D. (2000) Advances in spermatogonial stem cell transplantation. *Rev. Reprod.* 5:183-188.

Jung, Y.H., Gupta, M.K., Oh, S.H., Uhm, S.J., and Lee, H.T. (2010a) Glial cell line-derived neurotrophic factor alters the growth characteristics and genomic imprinting of mouse multipotent adult germline stem cells. *Exp. Cell Res.* 316:747-761.

Jung, Y.H., Gupta, M.K., Shin, J.Y., Uhm, S.J., and Lee, H.T. (2010b) MicroRNA signature in testes-derived male germ-line stem cells. *Mol. Hum. Reprod.* 16:804-810.

Kanatsu-Shinohara, M., Inoue, K., Lee, J., Miki, H., Ogonuki, N., Toyokuni, S., Ogura, A., and Shinohara, T. (2006) Anchorage-independent growth of mouse male germline stem cells in vitro. *Biol. Reprod.* 74:522-529.

Kanatsu-Shinohara, M., Inoue, K., Lee, J., Yoshimoto, M., Ogonuki, N., Miki, H., Baba, S., Kato, T., Kazuki, Y., Toyokuni, S., Toyoshima, M., Niwa, O., Oshimura, M., Heike, T., Nakahata, T., Ishino, F., Ogura, A., and Shinohara, T. (2004a) Generation of pluripotent stem cells from neonatal mouse testis. *Cell* 119:1001-1012.

Kanatsu-Shinohara, M., Inoue, K., Ogonuki, N., Miki, H., Yoshida, S., Toyokuni, S., Lee, J., Ogura, A., and Shinohara, T. (2007) Leukemia inhibitory factor enhances formation of germ cell colonies in neonatal mouse testis culture. *Biol. Reprod.* 76:55-62.

Kanatsu-Shinohara, M., Lee, J., Inoue, K., Ogonuki, N., Miki, H., Toyokuni, S., Ikawa, M., Nakamura, T., Ogura, A., and Shinohara, T. (2008) Pluripotency of a single spermatogonial stem cell in mice. *Biol. Reprod.* 78:681-687.

Kanatsu-Shinohara, M., Ogonuki, N., Inoue, K., Miki, H., Ogura, A., Toyokuni, S., and Shinohara, T. (2003) Long-term proliferation in culture and germline transmission of mouse male germline stem cells. *Biol. Reprod.* 69:612-616.

Kanatsu-Shinohara, M., Toyokuni, S., and Shinohara, T. (2004b) CD9 is a surface marker on mouse and rat male germline stem cells. *Biol. Reprod.* 70:70-75.

Kee, K., Angeles, V.T., Flores, M., Nguyen, H.N., and Reijo Pera, R.A. (2009) Human DAZL, DAZ and BOULE genes modulate primordial germ-cell and haploid gamete formation. *Nature* 462:222-225.

Kiger, A.A., White-Cooper, H., and Fuller, M.T. (2000) Somatic support cells restrict germline stem cell self-renewal and promote differentiation. *Nature* 407:750-754.

Ko, K., Tapia, N., Wu, G., Kim, J.B., Bravo, M.J., Sasse, P., Glaser, T., Ruau, D., Han, D.W., Greber, B., Hausdorfer, K., Sebastiano, V., Stehling, M., Fleischmann, B.K., Brustle, O., Zenke, M., and Scholer, H.R. (2009) Induction of pluripotency in adult unipotent germline stem cells. *Cell Stem Cell* 5:87-96.

Koshimizu, U., Watanabe, D., Tajima, Y., and Nishimune, Y. (1992) Effects of W (c-kit) gene mutation on gametogenesis in male mice: agametic tubular segments in Wf/Wf testes. *Development* 114:861-867.

Kubota, H., Avarbock, M.R., and Brinster, R.L. (2003) Spermatogonial stem cells share some, but not all, phenotypic and functional characteristics with other stem cells. *Proc. Natl. Acad. Sci. USA* 100:6487-6492.

Kubota, H., Avarbock, M.R., and Brinster, R.L. (2004a) Culture conditions and single growth factors affect fate determination of mouse spermatogonial stem cells. *Biol. Reprod.* 71:722-731.

Kubota, H., Avarbock, M.R., and Brinster, R.L. (2004b) Growth factors essential for self-renewal and expansion of mouse spermatogonial stem cells. *Proc. Natl. Acad. Sci. USA* 101:16489-16494.

Lee, J., Kanatsu-Shinohara, M., Inoue, K., Ogonuki, N., Miki, H., Toyokuni, S., Kimura, T., Nakano, T., Ogura, A., and Shinohara, T. (2007) Akt mediates self-renewal division of mouse spermatogonial stem cells. *Development* 134:1853-1859.

Lin, L.F., Doherty, D.H., Lile, J.D., Bektesh, S., and Collins, F. (1993) GDNF: a glial cell line-derived neurotrophic factor for midbrain dopaminergic neurons. *Science* 260:1130-1132.

Linher, K., Wu, D., and Li, J. (2007) Glial cell line-derived neurotrophic factor: an intraovarian factor that enhances oocyte developmental competence in vitro. *Endocrinology* 148:4292-4301.

Meng, X., Lindahl, M., Hyvonen, M.E., Parvinen, M., de Rooij, D.G., Hess, M.W., Raatikainen-Ahokas, A., Sainio, K., Rauvala, H., Lakso, M., Pichel, J.G., Westphal, H., Saarma, M., and Sariola, H. (2000) Regulation of cell fate decision of undifferentiated spermatogonia by GDNF. *Science* 287:1489-1493.

Mullaney, B.P., and Skinner, M.K. (1993) Transforming growth factor-beta (beta 1, beta 2, and beta 3) gene expression and action during pubertal development of the seminiferous tubule: potential role at the onset of spermatogenesis. *Mol. Endocrinol.* 7:67-76.

Nakagawa, T., Nabeshima, Y., and Yoshida, S. (2007) Functional identification of the actual and potential stem cell compartments in mouse spermatogenesis. *Dev. Cell* 12:195-206.

Nakagawa, T., Sharma, M., Nabeshima, Y., Braun, R.E., and Yoshida, S. (2010) Functional hierarchy and reversibility within the murine spermatogenic stem cell compartment. *Science* 328:62-67.

Nayernia, K., Nolte, J., Michelmann, H.W., Lee, J.H., Rathsack, K., Drusenheimer, N., Dev, A., Wulf, G., Ehrmann, I.E., Elliott, D.J., Okpanyi, V., Zechner, U., Haaf, T., Meinhardt, A., and Engel, W. (2006) In vitro-differentiated embryonic stem cells give rise to male gametes that can generate offspring mice. *Dev. Cell* 11:125-132.

Oakberg, E.F. (1971) Spermatogonial stem-cell renewal in the mouse. *Anat. Rec.* 169:515-531.

Oatley, J.M., Avarbock, M.R., and Brinster, R.L. (2007) Glial cell line-derived neurotrophic factor regulation of genes essential for self-renewal of mouse spermatogonial stem cells is dependent on Src family kinase signaling. *J. Biol. Chem.* 282:25842-25851.

Oatley, J.M., Avarbock, M.R., Telaranta, A.I., Fearon, D.T., and Brinster, R.L. (2006) Identifying genes important for spermatogonial stem cell self-renewal and survival. *Proc. Natl. Acad. Sci. USA* 103:9524-9529.

Oatley, J.M., Oatley, M.J., Avarbock, M.R., Tobias, J.W., and Brinster, R.L. (2009) Colony stimulating factor 1 is an extrinsic stimulator of mouse spermatogonial stem cell self-renewal. *Development* 136:1191-1199.

Ogawa, T., Dobrinski, I., Avarbock, M.R., and Brinster, R.L. (2000) Transplantation of male germ line stem cells restores fertility in infertile mice. *Nat. Med.* 6:29-34.

Oh, S.H., Jung, Y.H., Gupta, M.K., Uhm, S.J., and Lee, H.T. (2009) H19 gene is epigenetically stable in mouse multipotent germline stem cells. *Mol. Cells* 27:635-640.

Ohbo, K., Yoshida, S., Ohmura, M., Ohneda, O., Ogawa, T., Tsuchiya, H., Kuwana, T., Kehler, J., Abe, K., Scholer, H.R., and Suda, T. (2003) Identification and characterization of stem cells in prepubertal spermatogenesis in mice small star, filled. *Dev. Biol.* 258:209-225.

Ortega, S., Ittmann, M., Tsang, S.H., Ehrlich, M., and Basilico, C. (1998) Neuronal defects and delayed wound healing in mice lacking fibroblast growth factor 2. *Proc. Natl. Acad. Sci. USA* 95:5672-5677.

Orwig, K.E., Shinohara, T., Avarbock, M.R., and Brinster, R.L. (2002) Functional analysis of stem cells in the adult rat testis. *Biol. Reprod.* 66:944-949.

Petersen, C., and Soder, O. (2006) The sertoli cell--a hormonal target and 'super' nurse for germ cells that determines testicular size. *Horm. Res.* 66:153-161.

Rassoulzadegan, M., Paquis-Flucklinger, V., Bertino, B., Sage, J., Jasin, M., Miyagawa, K., van Heyningen, V., Besmer, P., and Cuzin, F. (1993) Transmeiotic differentiation of male germ cells in culture. *Cell* 75:997-1006.

Richardson, L.L., Kleinman, H.K., and Dym, M. (1995) Basement membrane gene expression by Sertoli and peritubular myoid cells in vitro in the rat. *Biol. Reprod.* 52:320-330.

Ryu, B.Y., Kubota, H., Avarbock, M.R., and Brinster, R.L. (2005) Conservation of spermatogonial stem cell self-renewal signaling between mouse and rat. *Proc. Natl. Acad. Sci. USA* 102:14302-14307.

Sada, A., Suzuki, A., Suzuki, H., and Saga, Y. (2009) The RNA-binding protein NANOS2 is required to maintain murine spermatogonial stem cells. *Science* 325:1394-1398.

Sadri-Ardekani, H., Mizrak, S.C., van Daalen, S.K., Korver, C.M., Roepers-Gajadien, H.L., Koruji, M., Hovingh, S., de Reijke, T.M., de la Rosette, J.J., van der Veen, F., de Rooij, D.G., Repping, S., and van Pelt, A.M. (2009) Propagation of human spermatogonial stem cells in vitro. *Jama* 302:2127-2134.

Sakai, N. (2002) Transmeiotic differentiation of zebrafish germ cells into functional sperm in culture. *Development* 129:3359-3365.

Sariola, H., and Saarma, M. (2003) Novel functions and signalling pathways for GDNF. *J. Cell Sci.* 116:3855-3862.

Schofield, R. (1978) The relationship between the spleen colony-forming cell and the haemopoietic stem cell. *Blood Cells* 4:7-25.

Schrans-Stassen, B.H., Saunders, P.T., Cooke, H.J., and de Rooij, D.G. (2001) Nature of the spermatogenic arrest in Dazl -/- mice. *Biol. Reprod.* 65:771-776.

Schrans-Stassen, B.H., van de Kant, H.J., de Rooij, D.G., and van Pelt, A.M. (1999) Differential expression of c-kit in mouse undifferentiated and differentiating type A spermatogonia. *Endocrinology* 140:5894-5900.

Seandel, M., James, D., Shmelkov, S.V., Falciatori, I., Kim, J., Chavala, S., Scherr, D.S., Zhang, F., Torres, R., Gale, N.W., Yancopoulos, G.D., Murphy, A., Valenzuela, D.M., Hobbs, R.M., Pandolfi, P.P., and Rafii, S. (2007) Generation of functional multipotent adult stem cells from GPR125+ germline progenitors. *Nature* 449:346-350.

Shinohara, T., Orwig, K.E., Avarbock, M.R., and Brinster, R.L. (2000) Spermatogonial stem cell enrichment by multiparameter selection of mouse testis cells. *Proc. Natl. Acad. Sci. USA* 97:8346-8351.

Shinohara, T., Orwig, K.E., Avarbock, M.R., and Brinster, R.L. (2001) Remodeling of the postnatal mouse testis is accompanied by dramatic changes in stem cell number and niche accessibility. *Proc. Natl. Acad. Sci. USA* 98:6186-6191.

Shuttlesworth, G.A., de Rooij, D.G., Huhtaniemi, I., Reissmann, T., Russell, L.D., Shetty, G., Wilson, G., and Meistrich, M.L. (2000) Enhancement of A spermatogonial proliferation and differentiation in irradiated rats by gonadotropin-releasing hormone antagonist administration. *Endocrinology* 141:37-49.

Sicinski, P., Donaher, J.L., Geng, Y., Parker, S.B., Gardner, H., Park, M.Y., Robker, R.L., Richards, J.S., McGinnis, L.K., Biggers, J.D., Eppig, J.J., Bronson, R.T., Elledge, S.J., and Weinberg, R.A. (1996) Cyclin D2 is an FSH-responsive gene involved in gonadal cell proliferation and oncogenesis. *Nature* 384:470-474.

Simon, L., Ekman, G.C., Tyagi, G., Hess, R.A., Murphy, K.M., and Cooke, P.S. (2007) Common and distinct factors regulate expression of mRNA for ETV5 and GDNF, Sertoli cell proteins essential for spermatogonial stem cell maintenance. *Exp. Cell Res.* 313:3090-3099.

Sunters, A., Thomas, D.P., Yeudall, W.A., and Grigoriadis, A.E. (2004) Accelerated cell cycle progression in osteoblasts overexpressing the c-fos proto-oncogene: induction of cyclin A and enhanced CDK2 activity. *J. Biol. Chem.* 279:9882-9891.

Swan, S.H., Elkin, E.P., and Fenster, L. (2000) The question of declining sperm density revisited: an analysis of 101 studies published 1934-1996. *Environ. Health Perspect.* 108:961-966.

Tadokoro, Y., Yomogida, K., Ohta, H., Tohda, A., and Nishimune, Y. (2002) Homeostatic regulation of germinal stem cell proliferation by the GDNF/FSH pathway. *Mech. Dev.* 113:29-39.

Tascou, S., Nayernia, K., Samani, A., Schmidtke, J., Vogel, T., Engel, W., and Burfeind, P. (2000) Immortalization of murine male germ cells at a discrete stage of differentiation by a novel directed promoter-based selection strategy. *Biol. Reprod.* 63:1555-1561.

Tegelenbosch, R.A., and de Rooij, D.G. (1993) A quantitative study of spermatogonial multiplication and stem cell renewal in the C3H/101 F1 hybrid mouse. *Mutat. Res.* 290:193-200.

Toyooka, Y., Tsunekawa, N., Akasu, R., and Noce, T. (2003) Embryonic stem cells can form germ cells in vitro. *Proc. Natl. Acad. Sci. USA* 100:11457-11462.

Tsutsui, T., Hesabi, B., Moons, D.S., Pandolfi, P.P., Hansel, K.S., Koff, A., and Kiyokawa, H. (1999) Targeted disruption of CDK4 delays cell cycle entry with enhanced p27(Kip1) activity. *Mol. Cell Biol.* 19:7011-7019.

van Pelt, A.M., Morena, A.R., van Dissel-Emiliani, F.M., Boitani, C., Gaemers, I.C., de Rooij, D.G., and Stefanini, M. (1996) Isolation of the synchronized A spermatogonia from adult vitamin A-deficient rat testes. *Biol. Reprod.* 55:439-444.

Watt, F.M., and Hogan, B.L. (2000) Out of Eden: stem cells and their niches. *Science* 287:1427-1430.

Wellik, D.M., Hawkes, P.J., and Capecchi, M.R. (2002) Hox11 paralogous genes are essential for metanephric kidney induction. *Genes Dev.* 16:1423-1432.

Yomogida, K., Yagura, Y., Tadokoro, Y., and Nishimune, Y. (2003) Dramatic expansion of germinal stem cells by ectopically expressed human glial cell line-derived neurotrophic factor in mouse Sertoli cells. *Biol. Reprod.* 69:1303-1307.

Yoon, K.A., Chae, Y.M., and Cho, J.Y. (2009) FGF2 stimulates SDF-1 expression through the Erm transcription factor in Sertoli cells. *J. Cell Physiol.* 220:245-256.

Yoshida, S., Sukeno, M., and Nabeshima, Y. (2007) A vasculature-associated niche for undifferentiated spermatogonia in the mouse testis. *Science* 317:1722-1726.

Yoshida, S., Takakura, A., Ohbo, K., Abe, K., Wakabayashi, J., Yamamoto, M., Suda, T., and Nabeshima, Y. (2004) Neurogenin3 delineates the earliest stages of spermatogenesis in the mouse testis. *Dev. Biol.* 269:447-458.

Yu, Z., Guo, R., Ge, Y., Ma, J., Guan, J., Li, S., Sun, X., Xue, S., and Han, D. (2003) Gene expression profiles in different stages of mouse spermatogenic cells during spermatogenesis. *Biol. Reprod.* 69:37-47.

Yu, Z., Ji, P., Cao, J., Zhu, S., Li, Y., Zheng, L., Chen, X., and Feng, L. (2009) Dazl promotes germ cell differentiation from embryonic stem cells. *J. Mol. Cell Biol.* 1:93-103.

Zechner, U., Nolte, J., Wolf, M., Shirneshan, K., Hajj, N.E., Weise, D., Kaltwasser, B., Zovoilis, A., Haaf, T., and Engel, W. (2009) Comparative methylation profiles and telomerase biology of mouse multipotent adult germline stem cells and embryonic stem cells. *Mol. Hum. Reprod.* 15:345-353.

Zhang, C., Yeh, S., Chen, Y.T., Wu, C.C., Chuang, K.H., Lin, H.Y., Wang, R.S., Chang, Y.J., Mendis-Handagama, C., Hu, L., Lardy, H., and Chang, C. (2006a) Oligozoospermia with normal fertility in male mice lacking the androgen receptor in testis peritubular myoid cells. *Proc. Natl. Acad. Sci. USA* 103:17718-17723.

Zhang, X., Ebata, K.T., Robaire, B., and Nagano, M.C. (2006b) Aging of male germ line stem cells in mice. *Biol. Reprod.* 74:119-124.

Zovoilis, A., Nolte, J., Drusenheimer, N., Zechner, U., Hada, H., Guan, K., Hasenfuss, G., Nayernia, K., and Engel, W. (2008) Multipotent adult germline stem cells and embryonic stem cells have similar microRNA profiles. *Mol. Hum. Reprod.* 14:521-529.

In: In Vitro Fertilization
Editor: Samantha P. Steiger, pp.165-176
ISBN 978-1-61209-961-3

Chapter IX

OMICS Techniques in Human Embryo Viability Assessment

***Roseli Fernandes Gonçalves*[*1], *Andrea Giannotti Galuppo*[≠2] *and Gary J. Killian*[3]**

[1]Department of Animal Reproduction, College of Veterinary Medicine and Animal Sciences, São Paulo University, São Paulo, SP, Brazil
[2]Embryology and Animal Reproduction Biotech Laboratory, College of Veterinary Medicine, Rio Grande do Sul Federal University, Porto Alegre, RS, Brazil
[3]National Wildlife Research Center, USDA – APHIS, CO, USA

Abstract

OMICS technologies (genomic, transcriptomic, proteinomic, metabolomic, and lipidomic) in principle allow visualization of changes that take place when the genetics, nutrition or environment of an organism is altered. Targeted compositional analysis is a valuable tool of assisted reproduction which enables quantitative analysis of biomarkers associated with oocyte and embryo viability. Contemporary embryo assessment strategies are largely based on embryo morphology and cleavage rate. While these systems have been successful in improving pregnancy rates and reducing multiple gestations, their precision is still insufficient. The present chapter describes the current status of embryo assessment techniques for human *in vitro* fertilization and discusses the potential use of OMICS technologies as a predictor of embryo viability.

[*] Department of Animal Reproduction, College of Veterinary Medicine and Animal Sciences, São Paulo University, São Paulo, SP, Brazil; Telephone: 55 - 11- 30917914; Fax: 55 - 11 – 30917412.

[≠] Embryology and Animal Reproduction Biotech Laboratory, College of Veterinary Medicine, Rio Grande do Sul Federal University, Porto Alegre, RS, Brazil; Telephone: 55 - 51 - 33086126; Fax: 55 - 51 -33087305.

Introduction

In assisted reproductive technology (ART), pregnancy and birth rates following in vitro fertilization (IVF) attempts remain low. Indeed, 2 out of 3 IVF cycles fail to result in pregnancy (SART, 2004) and more than 8 out of 10 transferred embryos fail to implant (Kovalevsky and Patrizio, 2005).

The selection of embryos with higher implantation potential has been one of the major challenges in ART. This selection is currently based on morphological criteria such as growth rate, early cleavage on day-1, degree of fragmentation, and blastocyst formation (Ebner et al., 2003). However, the predictive power of this approach is still limited. With the emergence of new technologies like 'omics', there are new biomarkers as discovery tools that can be applied to IVF for oocyte and/or embryo selection (Hillier, 2008).

The term "omics" can be considered as a neologism that designates broad fields of biology with a name that end with the suffix "omes". This term probably has its origins in the world biomes in the late 20th century and became very popular with the large study of the total human and other organisms genes, called genome. The "omic" approaches propose a global characterization of specific classes of target biomolecules in uni or multi-cellular systems as a strategy to achieve comprehensive understanding of biological functions. The "omics revolution" is closely related to recent technical revolutions in mass spectrometry (MS). MS is a rapidly expanding technique in both industry and academia. It is widely and routinely used for biomolecules analysis aimed at drug discovery, diagnostics, and comprehensive assessment of biological, physiological, and pathological conditions (Griffiths and Wang, 2009). In this review, we will describe the current status of embryo assessment techniques for human *in vitro* fertilization and discusses the potential use of OMICS technologies as a predictor of embryo viability.

Genomic Assessment of Viability in Assisted Reproduction

The genomics, aimed at performing the entire genetic sequencing of organisms, represented the seminal step towards the understanding of the complex logic that orchestrates the function of all organisms or the defects leading to diseases (Stratton *et al.*, 2009; Shuldiner and Pollin, 2010). However to express the phenotype, information needs to flow from DNA via carrier biomolecules through processes that have being addressed by new "omic" sciences such as the transcriptomics, proteomics, metabolomics, glycomics, lipidomics, fluxomics and interactomics.

While DNA sequence analysis is not a likely strategy for embryo viability assessment, chromosome numbers and integrity have been successfully investigated as a determinant of embryo viability. The number of chromosomes in the embryo has been analyzed in an effort to increase IVF success by identifying and excluding aneuploid embryos. The analysis is invasive and requires biopsy of blastomere(s) or trophoectoderm from the embryo, 3 or 5 days after fertilization, respectively. Alternatively, removal of the polar body extruded from the oocyte during meiosis has been performed to test for oocyte aneuploidy. It is noteworthy that when embryo is biopsied on day 5 after fertilization followed by analysis, fresh embryo transfer cannot be performed and cryopreservation and transfer in a subsequent cycle becomes necessary (Hassold and Hunt, 2001; Staessen et al., 2008; Northrop et al., 2010).

These approaches have recently been categorized as preimplantation genetic screening (PGS) by the European Society for Human Reproduction and embryology (ESHRE) to distinguish them from preimplantation genetic diagnosis (PGD), performed for patients that are at high risk of transmitting a genetic or chromosomal abnormality to their children, which include single gene defects (autosomal dominant, autosomal recessive, X-linked disorders) and chromosomal abnormalities (translocations, inversions, etc.) (Thornhill *et al.*, 2005).

Trancriptomic Analysis of Viability in Assisted Reproduction

Transcriptomics aimed to perform the study of all set of RNA molecules (mRNA, rRNA, tRNA and non-coding RNA) in a single cell or organism (Blow, 2009). How transcriptomics reflects the genes that have being active expressed at given time in the cell, it is also referred as expression profiling. The main technique used to address this "omic" approach is the RNA and DNA microarray.

Transcriptome analysis within the context of gametes and embryos can serve different purposes. It can be used to address the phenotype of a cell in order to understand a physiological process, mainly done in a research environment with animal or human samples, or it can be used for diagnostic purposes where the goal is to select either the best oocyte/embryo or to assess the hormonal stimulation response (Assou *et al.*, 2008, Hamel, et al., 2008). Most normal somatic tissues are easier to analyze than embryos, mainly because they are more abundant and their RNA is a more direct representation of the protein content that drives the phenotype of the cell.

The perception that cumulus cells (CC) have a central role in the communication of signals within the follicle and in the support of oocyte maturation has led various groups to focus their research on the analysis of CC gene expression, in the hunt for novel markers of oocyte competence and pregnancy outcome. There are no reviews yet on the use of follicular markers or cumulus markers as this field is still in its infancy, but several papers have found associations between specific markers and either embryo quality. Several of these markers are actually being validated in larger clinical trials to assess their predictive value. The first challenge of those clinical trials is finding markers that will remain valid in all sorts of genetic backgrounds, hormonal treatments and clinical conditions. The second challenge is related to creating a robust process to assess the level of a given marker or a combination of them in a clinical environment. To achieve such robustness, it may be required that specific proteins translated from unique RNA are measured instead of the RNA itself to minimize the risk of degradation as RNA is a very sensitive molecule compared to DNA or proteins and requires very careful handling procedures (Fragouli *et al*, 2007; Gasca *et al*, 2007; Cillo *et al*, 2007; Feuerstein *et al*, 2007; Van Montfoort *et al*, 2008; Hamel *et al*, 2008; Assou *et al*, 2008; Wells *et al*, 2008; Huang and Wells, 2010; Kwon *et al*, 2010).

Oocytes and early embryos require additional considerations to prevent aberrant transcriptomic results. It is most problematic when different stage embryos are compared, considering that the number and size of the cells they contain are dramatically different and that their transcriptional and translational activity evolves prior and after the maternal to embryonic transition. The comparison of fixed numbers of embryos at different stages will lead to an amplification bias. Indeed, sample with the same number of embryos at different stages will contain different amounts of material, making comparison irrelevant. The comparison of fixed amount of material will also be physiologically questionable since the end point values will be comparing different numbers of embryos. The scarcity of this type of biological material necessitates the use of a global amplification method to yield sufficient material for downstream transcriptomic study. As such, PCR based methods have been mostly discarded, as they are known to lead to a plateau phase, which can disrupt the relative abundance of RNA within a sample. As a consequence, linear methods based on in vitro transcription have taken the forefront of sample amplification. It has recently been shown that these methods, although mostly linear, also reach a plateau phase, which homogenizes the reaction's output (Gilbert, *et al.*2009). This leads to an important distortion in the natural differences in RNA contents between distinct developmental stages, failing to account for such important bias may lead to false discoveries.

Proteomic Analysis of Viability in Assisted Reproduction

Proteomics is, together with genomics, the most well know "omic" approach (Cravatt *et al*, 2007). The proteomics era is coincident with significant developments in mass spectrometry (MS), as well as fast bioinformatics tools, database search engines, and fulfillment of genome sequencing efforts. Proteomics involves not only the identification of gene products and their abundances, but also the use of protein interactions for analysis of protein complexes, protein-protein interaction networks, and the dynamic behavior of the networks as a function of time or experimental condition. The major breakthrough of MS-based proteomics for biomarker search is the possibility to quantify a wide spectrum of proteins, and the easiness of assembling multiplex detection in a single measurement, an approach believed to lead personalized medicine and treatments in the future (Pan *et al*, 2009).

Proteins translated from RNA transcripts are directly responsible for cellular function. Gene expression studies of these RNA transcripts, though valuable, have been shown to often not predict protein abundance or function. Several mechanisms, including targeted mRNA degradation and protein degradation, can be utilized by the cell during regulation of transcription/translation resulting in a lack of association between gene expression, RNA transcripts and protein expression. Consequently, in order to understand cellular function and comprehend biological processes and/or disease states, a depth investigation of the mammalian proteome is vital. Proteomics involves not only the identification of gene products and their abundances, but also the use of protein interactomes for analysis of protein complexes, protein-protein interaction networks, and the dynamic behavior of the networks as a function of time or experimental condition (Pan *et al*, 2009).

MS has rapidly become an important technology in proteomic profiling. MS involves an ion source for production of a charged species in the gas phase, and an analyzer, which can separate ions by their mass-to-charge (m/z) ratio. Several commonly used ionization methods include electrospray ionization and surface-enhanced laser desorption/ionization (SELDI), which are coupled to time-of-flight (TOF), ion trap or quadrupole analyzers. SELDITOF MS, with specific capture affinity protein chips, has allowed fast, cost-effective, high-throughput analysis of small sample volumes (microliter range) and enables sensitivity to be in the picomole to femtomole range (Pan *et al*, 2009). Bound proteins are laser activated thereby liberating gaseous ions by desorption/ionization. The TOF tube is under a vacuum which causes smaller ions to travel faster towards the detector thereby allowing a separation of these ions according tom/z ratio represented as a protein profile (Seibert et al., 2004). Identification of proteins following MS profiling is typically performed by protease digestion generating distinct cleavage products identifiable by tandem MS analysis and protein database searching (Liebler, 2002).

MS proteomics analysis in embryos has been recently reported for porcine (Sutovsky *et al*, 2005), mouse (Katz-Jaffe *et al*, 2006a), human (Katz-Jaffe *et al*, 2006b, 2009), bringing new information regarding protein profile as a function of oxygen concentration during embryo in vitro culture and between different stages of development. In ART, the proteome is of particular interest in non-invasive gamete and embryo assessment by means of the secretome, like those proteins produced by cells and secreted in the culture medium (Hathout, 2007). As for the embryo proteome, a recent review stated that despite new advances in proteomic technologies, knowledge of the proteome of the mammalian preimplantation embryo (including mouse, porcine, rabbit and human) remains limited. It was concluded that the combined effect of limited template, low protein expression and the lack of sensitivity of proteomics platforms are the main hurdles (Katz-Jaffe and Gardner, 2007).

It is clear that protein analysis should be the preferred end point of all physiological analyses. Unfortunately, very few publications are displaying even a partial protein pattern for ovarian cells (Wang *et al.*, 2009). Follicular fluid is considered an interesting target for "omic" techniques in ART, especially proteomics, since it represents the natural microenvironment for oocytes during maturation and embryo development. Several publications have identified a number of proteins in this fluid and it has recently become a target for the identification of protein markers associated either with disease (Atiomo, et al., 2009), or oocyte of higher quality (Jarkovska *et al*, 2010). One of the challenges that scientists face with follicular fluid is the abundance of albumin, immunoglobulin and other abundant proteins present in serum.

In proteomic analysis of culture medium, which is different from metabolomic studies, most of the metabolites will be peptide chains that do not form functional proteins. Some studies have proposed that viable embryos possess a unique proteome and that some of these proteins are potentially secreted into the surrounding culture medium, contributing to the "secretome" (Katz-Jaffe *et al*, 2006b, 2009). One of the earliest studies of the human embryonic secretome revealed the release of platelet activating factor (PAF), a soluble factor (not a protein) that is produced and secreted by mammalian preimplantation embryos (O'Neill, 2005). PAF release causes a range of alterations in maternal physiology, including platelet activation, changes in uterine tube, endometrial and maternal immune functions. PAF also acts in an autocrine fashion as a trophic/survival factor for the early embryo. In vitro, supplementation of culture medium with PAF improves embryo development (O'Neill, 2005).

Katz-Jaffe, using SELDI-TOF-MS (Surface-enhanced laser desorption/ionization time of flight mass spectrometer), identified different secretome profiles for each stage of embryonic development. Recently, a study using protein micro-arrays that contained 120 protein targets was used to simultaneously compare two given conditions. This system has a detection limit of 10–250 000 pg/ml. They collected conditioned media from human embryos (implanted and non-implanted) before their transfer using a single embryo transfer program. Interestingly, proteins like CXCL13 (BCL, B lymphocyte chemoattractant), stem cell factor (SCF), and macrophage-stimulating protein-a (MSP-a) significantly ($P < .005$) decreased and were, therefore, consumed by the human blastocyst. In contrast, soluble tumor necrosis factor (TNF) receptor 1 (sTNFR1) significantly increased in the media where the blastocyst was present in comparison with the control media. Unfortunately none of the proteins investigated was significantly upregulated/secreted by the implanted blastocyst (Dominguez *et al.*, 2008).

Metabolomic Analysis of Viability in Assisted Reproduction

Metabolomics aim to study changes of the higher number possible of different small-molecules metabolites in a cell, tissue, organ or organism (Carroll *et al*, 2010; Zhao *et al*, 2010). Differently from transcriptomics and proteomics, metabolomics profiling can give a snapshot of the physiology of the cell and have been used widely nowadays.

Cells produce a innumerable of metabolites, which are the functional end products of all biological processes, and therefore a promising form of non-invasive methods for embryo selection in the ART field. Metabolomics analysis approaches are aimed at identifying and quantifying target intracellular metabolites usually with MW lower than 1.000 Da, and have traditionally used techniques such as nuclear magnetic resonance (NMR) and fourier transform infrared spectroscopy (FTIR; Katz-Jaffe *et al*, 2009). Nonetheless, due to the unmatched combination of speed, sensitivity and selectivity. MS approaches are becoming the most important techniques in current metabolomics studies.

Relevant information regarding oocyte and embryo viability has used targeted metabolomic approaches for amino acids analysis using conventional chromatrography (Houghton *et al*, 2002). Proper metabolic turnover is essential for a pre-implantation embryo to remain viable and develop into a successful pregnancy. Consequently, nutrients and metabolites within the culture environment have been studied as potential predictors of embryo viability. A key aspect of pre-implantation embryo development is the switch from carboxylic acid to glucose metabolism, which occurs around the time of pre- and post-compaction, and is among the best characterized phenomena of embryonic metabolic regulation (Leese, 1995). The turnover of three amino acids in human embryos culture medium (asparagines, glycine and leucine) was correlated with pregnancy and live birth, which in turn were not associated with maternal age and embryo cell number or morphological grading (Brison *et al*, 2004).

The capacity to metabolize glucose increases significantly at the transition from the morula to blastocyst stage and also seems to reflect the embryo's developmental potential and viability (Devreker, 2007). Gardner and Leese (1987) measured glucose uptake by microfluorescence in Day 4 mouse blastocysts prior to embryo transfer. Embryos that resulted in term pregnancies had a significantly higher glucose uptake in culture than embryos that failed to progress. Gardner *et al.* (2001) also reported that the glucose consumption by Day 4 human embryos was higher in embryos that formed blastocysts and correlated with morphologic grade. More recently, Urbanski *et al.* reported the development of a microfluidics system that allows simultaneous measurement of pyruvate, lactate, and glucose in small volumes of mouse embryo culture media (Urbanski *et al.*, 2008). This report is encouraging, as it constitutes a major improvement in clinical applicability of metabolite measurement.

Using high performance liquid chromatography mass spectrometry (HPLCMS) Houghton *et al.* quantified secretion and uptake of amino acids by human embryos at different stages of pre-implantation development (Houghton *et al.*, 2002). They found that a lower uptake of glutamine, arginine, and methionine and a lower release of alanine and asparagine by day 2 and 3 embryos correlate with successful development to the blastocyct stage, whereas in 8-cell and morula stage embryos, blastocyst development is associated with lower uptake of serine and release of alanine and glycine. In all stages examined, lower amino acid turnover calculated by determining the sum of depletion and appearance of all amino acids, was associated with better development, consistent with the "quiet embryo" hypothesis (Leese *et al.*, 2008).

Brison et al. determined the changes in the concentrations of amino acids in spent human embryo culture media and identified amino acids that correlate with clinical pregnancy and live birth (Brison *et al.*, 2004). They found that a decrease in glycine and leucine and increase in asparagines levels in the culture medium correlate with clinical pregnancy and live birth (Brison, et al., 2004). Seli et al. used proton nuclear magnetic resonance (1H NMR) and found an association between higher glutamate levels in the culture media and clinical pregnancy and live birth (Seli *et al.*, 2008). In this study, embryos were cultured in 25 ml medium for 48 hours prior to transfer on day 3. The differences in the volume and type of culture medium used, length of culture, and technology used to measure amino acids may explain differences in identified amino acid biomarkers.

There are more than 25,000 genes in the human genome, encoding for approximately 100,000-200,000 transcripts, and 1 million proteins, whereas there may be as few as 2500-3000 metabolites that make up the human metabolome (Botros *et al.*, 2008). As the number of metabolites is significantly lower than the number of genes and proteins in a cell or organism, thorough metabolomic analysis can be achieved in a relatively faster period of time than genomics experiments. Nevertheless, metabolomic studies require a multidisciplinary team, from sample collection and preparation through analytical operations to processing of raw data and analysis of the processed data. Metabolomics uses spectroscopic/spectrometric and chromatographic Techniques as analytical technologies to investigate complex metabolic/metabolomic profiles of biological systems (Botros, et al., 2008). The analysis of biological fluids by spectroscopic technologies is termed "biospectroscopy". The scientific platform that incorporates both biospectroscopy and metabolic profiling is commonly referred to as "biospectroscopy-based metabolomics" or "BSM". Both non-optical and optical spectroscopies have been used as analytical technologies for BSM.

Seli and collaborators used Raman and NIR spectroscopies to analyze day 3 spent culture media of invidually cultured embryos with known outcome (Seli *et al*, 2007). In this study, mean spectrum of embryos that resulted in a pregnancy and live birth was compared to that of embryos that failed to implant, and spectral regions most predictive of pregnancy outcome were identified. Then, using algorithms based on these spectral regions, a viability score was calculated for each embryo. Authors found that the mean viability score of embryos that implanted and resulted in a live birth were significantly higher compared to those that failed to result in a pregnancy (Seli, et al., 2007). Raman and NIR spectroscopies achieved a sensitivity of 76.5% and 83.3%, and a specificity of 86% and 75%, respectively. Moreover, the test was rapid (less than 1 minute per sample) and required a very small sample volume (less than 15 μl).

The model developed in this initial study (Seli, et al., 2007) was then tested in a blinded trial (Scott *et al.*, 2008) using Raman spectroscopy to analyze day 3 and day 5 spent culture media collected at a different center, where embryos were cultured in a different type of culture medium, and a different volume. In this study, the viability scores of day 3 and day 5 embryos that resulted in a live birth were significantly higher compared to the viability scores of embryos that failed to implant. The initial studies described above were followed by studies with larger sample size from IVF centers that routinely perform single embryo transfer (SET; Seli *et al.*, 2010, Seli *et al.*, 2009, Vergouw *et al.*, 2008).

Lipidomic Analysis of Viability in Assisted Reproduction

Lipidomics aimed to perform the study of the complete profile of lipids produced in a biological system, respectively, also studying the pathways and networks involved in each specific class of compounds (Blanksby and Mitchell, 2010). Driving by the pivotal role of lipids in cell membrane structure and in cell signaling, the field of metabolomics has extended into lipidomics. The lipidoma from mammalian organisms are represented by a great variety of tens of thousands lipid species (Van Meer, 2005).

Two lipidomics protocols are mainly used, the use of selective extraction optimized for each lipid category, followed by their LC separation, and one that involves the direct MS analysis of lipid extracts without previous separation by selective extraction. MALDI-MS lipid fingerprinting of individual oocytes and embryos is a fast and high-throughput technique (Ferreira *et al*, 2010), which can add valuable information to experiments aimed at optimizing *in vitro* embryo culture systems for cryopreservation. Also the detection of the "ideal" lipid profiles obtained from *in vivo* derived embryos can be used as an indicative of embryo cryosensitivity.

Van Meer (2005) used MALDI-MS to obtain direct lipid fingerprinting of individual oocytes and embryos of various species. Due to the sensitivity and easiness of lipid ionization by MALDI, no sample extraction was needed. Embryos and oocytes were simply placed on a target plate, and covered with the MALDI matrix. PCs, SMs, and TAGs were detected in few seconds. Oocytes and embryos displayed different lipid profiles, and embryos cultured in low oxygen atmosphere (5%) and without fetal calf serum as a supplement, showed PCs with less palmitic acid (a saturated fatty acyl residue) and more oleic acid (an unsatured fatty acyl residue; Ferreira *et al*, 2010).

Conclusion

Between all the applications of "omics" techniques in human reproduction, the biomarker discovery field can be considered as the one with more development potential. Modern and powerful MS methods are revolutionizing the fields of proteomics, lipidomics and metabolomics. This MS revolution has encouraged researches to value the individual characterization and quantification of biomolecules in living systems, as well as the need of a systemic molecular biological view.

Preimplantation embryo development is one of the key features with implantation itself to achieve a pregnancy. Assisted Reproductive Technologies both in human and animal have improved our knowledge on these events, although it remains elusive to predict embryo potential to give a baby. Among various ways to define embryo viability, noninvasive approaches get a serious advantage linked to the final transfer of the embryo. "Omics" techniques devoted to characterize the embryo secretome using proteomic or metabolomic approaches may be non invasive. Based on a direct identification of products of the embryo metabolism or an assessment of profile(s) related with embryo viability, they have greatly improved their sensitivity to allow their use in clinical embryology, once validated. Oocyte-cumulus dialogue, as a key factor for oocyte competence to meiosis and embryo development, was particularly concerned with both genomic and proteomic assessment of cumulus cells. While it is not possible to designate at the time being which among these approaches will be robust and cost-efficient enough to help routinely the clinical embryologist in assisted reproductive techniques (ART), one can predict that our ability to select the ''right'' embryo will combine morphological criteria already available with validated biomarkers. Therefore, a fast, inexpensive, easy-to-use, and hopefully non-invasive test involving one or a combination of these parameters may soon be available in clinical practice.

References

Assou S, Haouzi D, Mahmoud K, Aouacheria A, Guillemin Y, Pantesco V, Rème T, Dechaud H, De Vos J and Hamamah S. A non-invasive test for assessing embryo potential by gene expression profiles of human cumulus cells: a proof of concept study. *Mol Hum Reprod* 2008;14:711-9.

Atiomo WU, Khalid S, Ziauddin A, Tooth D, Layfield R, Misiti S, Stigliano A, Borro M, Gentile G, Michienzi S et al. Framework for a systems approach to proteomic biomarker profiling in polycystic ovary syndrome. *Expert Rev* Proteomics 2009;6:469-99.

Blanksby SJ and Mitchell TW. Advances in mass spectrometry for lipidomics. *Annu Rev Anal Chem* 2010;3:433-465.

Botros L, Sakkas D,Seli E. Metabolomics and its application for non-invasive embryo assessment in IVF. . *Mol Hum Reprod* 2008;14:679-90.

Brison DR, Houghton FD, Falconer D, Roberts SA, Hawkhead J, Humpherson PG, Lieberman BA,Leese HJ. Identification of viable embryos in IVF by non-invasive measurement of amino acid trunover. *Hum Reprod* 2004;19:2319-24.

Carroll AJ, Badger MR, Harvey Millar A. The metabolome express project: enabling web-based processing, analysis and transparent dissemination of GC/MS metabolomics datasets. *BMC Bioinformatics* 2010;11:376.

Cillo F, Brevini TAL, Antonini S, Paffoni S, Ragni G, Gandolfi F. Association between human oocyte developmental competence and expression levels of some cumulus genes. *Reproduction* 2007;134:645-650.

Dominguez F, Gadea B, Esteban FJ, Horcajadas JA, Pellicer A,Simon C. Comparative protein-profile analysis of implanted versus non-implanted human blastocysts. *Hum Reprod* 2008;23:1993-2000.

Devreker F. Uptake and release of metabolites in human preimplantation embryos. In: Cohen J, Elder K (eds). *Human Preimplantation Embryo Selection*. London, UK: Taylor and Francis, 2007,325–336.

Ebner T, Moser M, Sommergruber M, Tews G. Selection based on morphological assessment of oocytes and embryos at different stages of preimplantation development: a review. *Hum Reprod Update* 2003;9:251-62.

Feuerstein P, Cadoret V, Dalbies-Tran R, Guerif F, Bidault R and Royere D. Gene expression in human cumulus cells: one approach to oocyte competence. *Hum Reprod* 2007;22:3069–3077.

Fragouli E, Bianchi V, Delhanty J, Patrizio P and Wells D. Gene expression analysis of human oocytes: Towards a non-invasive diagnosis of meiotic aneuploidy. *Hum Reprod* 2007;22(1) 70-78.

Gardner DK, Leese HJ. Assessment of embryo viability prior to transfer by the noninvasive measurement of glucose uptake. *J Exp Zool* 1987;242:103–105.

Gardner DK, Lane M, Stevens J, Schoolcraft WB. Noninvasive assessment of human embryo nutrient consumption as a measure of developmental potential. *Fertil Steril* 2001;76:1175–1180.

Gasca S, Pellestor F, Assou S, Loup V, Anahory T, Dechaud H, De Vos J, Hamamah S. Identifying new human oocyte marker genes: a microarray approach. *Reprod Biomed Online* 2007;14:175–183.

Gilbert I, Scantland S, Dufort I, Gordynska O, Labbe A, Sirard MA,Robert C. Real-time monitoring of aRNA production during T7 amplification to prevent the loss of sample representation during microarray hybridization sample preparation. *Nucleic Acids Res* 2009;37:e65.

Hamel M, Dufort I, Robert C, Gravel C, Leveille MC, Leader A, Sirard MA. Identification of differentially expressed markers in human follicular cells associated with competent oocytes. *Hum Reprod* 2008;23:1118–1127.

Griffiths WJ, Wang y. Mass spectrometry: from proteomics to metabolomics and lipidomics. *Chemical Soc Reviews* 2009;38(7):1882-1896.

Hassold T,Hunt P. To err (meiotically) is human: the genesis of human aneuploidy. *Nature Reviews Genetics* 2001;2:280-291.

Hillier SG. Research challenge: what is the best non-invasive test of oocyte/embryo competence? *Mol Hum Reprod* 2008;14:665.

Huang Z, Wells D. The human oocyte and cumulus cells relationship: new insights from the cumulus cell transcriptome. *Mol Hum Reprod* 2010;16(10):715-125.

Jarkovska K, Martinkova J, Liskova L, Halada P, Moos J, Rezabek K, Gadher SJ,Kovarova H. Proteome Mining of Human Follicular Fluid Reveals a Crucial Role of Complement Cascade and Key Biological Pathways in Women Undergoing in Vitro Fertilization. *J Proteome Res* 2010;9(3):1289-1301.

Katz-Jaffe MG, Gardner DK,Schoolcraft WB. Proteomic analysis of individual human embryos to identify novel biomarkers of development and viability. *Fertil Steril* 2006a;85:101-7.

Katz-Jaffe MG, Schoolcraft WB,Gardner DK. Analysis of protein expression (secretome) by human and mouse preimplantation embryos. *Fertil Steril* 2006b;86:678-85.

Katz-Jaffe MG,Gardner DK. Embryology in the era of proteomics. *Theriogenology* 2007;68(1):125-30.

Kovalevsky G, Patrizio P. High rates of embryo wastage with use of assisted reproductive technology: a look at the trends between 1995 and 2001 in the United States. *Fertil Steril* 2005;84:325–330.

Kwon H, Choi DH, Bae JH, Kim JH, Kim YS. mRNA expression pattern of insulin-like growth factor components of granulose cells and cumulus cells in women with and without polycystic ovary syndrome according to oocyte maturity. *Fertil Steril* 2010;94(6):2417-2420.

Leese HJ, Baumann CG, Brison DR, McEvoy TG,Sturmey RG. Metabolism of the viable mammalian embryo: quietness revisited. *Mol Hum Reprod* 2008;14:667-72.

Liebler DC. *Introduction to Proteomics: Tools for the New Biology*. Ottowa, New Jersey: Humana Press, 2002.

Northrop LE, Treff NRL, B.,Scott Jr. RT. Comprehensive microarray based aneuploidy screening demonstrates that cleavage stage fluorescence in situ hybridization (FISH) poorly predicts aneuploidy in embryos that develop to morphologically normal blastocysts. . 2010; *Mol Hum Reprod.*

O'Neill C. The role of paf in embryo physiology. *Hum Reprod Update* 2005;11:215-28.

Pan S, Aebersold R, Chen R, Rush J, Goodlett DR, McIntosh MW, Zhang J, Brentnall TA. Mass spectrometry based targeted protein quantification: methods and applications. *J Proteome Res* 2009;8(2):787-797.

Seibert V, Wiesner A, Buschmann T, Meuer J. Surface-enhanced laser desorption ionization time-of-flight mass spectrometry (SELDI TOF-MS) and ProteinChip technology in proteomics research. *Pathol Res Pract* 2004;200:83–94.

Seli E, Sakkas D, Scott R, Kwok JS, Rosendahl S,Burns DH. Non-Invasive metabolomic profiling of human embryo culture media using Raman and near infrared spectroscopy correlates with reproductive potential of embryos in women undergoing in vitro fertilization. *Fertil Steril* 2007;88:1350-7.

Seli E, Botros L, Sakkas D,Burns DH. Non-invasive metabolomic profiling of embryo culture media using proton NMR correlates with reproductive potential of embryos in women undergoing in vitro fertilization. *Fertil Steril* 2008;90:2183-2189.

Seli E, Vergouw CG, Morita H, Botros L, Roos P, Lambalk CB, Yamashita N, Kato O,Sakkas D. Non-invasive metabolomic profiling as an adjunct to morphology for non-invasive embryo assessment in women undergoing single embryo transfer. *Fertil Setil* 2009;94(2):535-542.

Seli E, Bruce C, Botros L, Henson M, Roos P, Judge K, Sakkas D,Group. atMS. Receiver Operating Characteristic (ROC) analysis of Day 5 morphology grading and metabolomic Viability Scores on predicting implantation outcome. *J Assist Reprod Genet* 2010; Epub.

Society for Assisted Reproductive Technology; American Society for Reproductive Medicine. Assisted reproductive technology in the United States: 2000 results generated from the American Society for Reproductive Medicine/Society for Assisted Reproductive Technology Registry. *Fertil Steril* 2004;81:1207–1220.

Staessen C, Verpoest W, Donoso P, Haentjens P, Van der Elst J, Liebaers I,Devroey P. Preimplantation genetic screening does not improve delivery rate in women under the age of 36 following single-embryo transfer. *Hum Reprod* 2008 23:2818-25.

Thornhill AR, deDie-Smulders CE, Geraedts JP, Harper JC, Harton GL, Lavery SA, Moutou C, Robinson MD, Schmutzler AG, Scriven PN et al. ESHRE PGD Consortium 'Best practice guidelines for clinical preimplantation genetic diagnosis (PGD) and preimplantation genetic screening (PGS)'. *Hum Reprod* 2005;20:35-48.

Urbanski JP, Johnson MT, Craig DD, Potter DL, Gardner DK,Thorsen T. Noninvasive metabolic profiling using microfluidics for analysis of single preimplantation embryos. *Anal Chem* 2008;80:6500-7.

Van Meer G. Cellular lipidomics. *Embo J* 2005;129(3):269-282.

Van Montfoort APA, Geraedts JPM, Dumoulin JCM, Stassen APM, Evers JLH, Ayoubi TAY. Differential gene expression in cumulus cells as a prognostic indicator of embryo viability: a microarray analysis. *Mol Hum Reprod* 2008;14:157–168.

Vergouw CG, Botros LL, Roos P, Lens JW, Schats R, Hompes PGA, Burns DH,Lambalk CB. Metabolomic profiling by near-infrared spectroscopy as a tool to assess embryo viability: a novel, non-invasive method for embryo selection. *Hum Reprod* 2008;23:1499-1504.

Wang N, Zhang P, Guo X, Xie J, Huo R, Wang F, Chen L, Shen J, Zhou Z, Shi Q, Zhao B, Sha J. Comparative proteome profile of immature rat ovary during primordial follicle assembly and development. *Proteomics* 2009;9:3425-34.

Wells D, Fragouli E, Bianchi V, Borini A and Patrizio P. Identification of novel non-invasive biomarkers of oocyte aneuploidy. *Fertil Steril* 2008;90(1), S35.

Zhao X, Fritsche J, Wang J, Chen J, Rittig K, Schmitt-Kopplin P, Fritsche A, Häring hU, Schleicher ED, Xu G, Lehmann R. Metabolomic fingerprints of fasting plasma and spot urine reveal human pre-diabetic metabolomic traits. *Metabolomics* 2010;6:362-374.

Index

B

C

D

E

F

G

H

I

J

K

L

M

N

O

P

Q

R

T

U

V

W

X

Y

Z